D0805816

not on our street

Pion Limited, 207 Brondesbury Park, London NW2 5JN

ISBN 0 85086 096 2

Printed in Great Britain by Page Bros (Norwich) Limited

not on our street
community attitudes
to mental health care

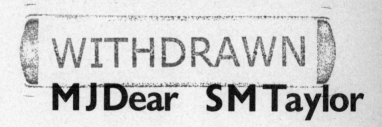

MJDear SMTaylor

Research in Planning and Design

Series editor Allen J Scott

p Pion Limited, 207 Brondesbury Park, London NW2 5JN

Preface

This book is about public attitudes toward the mentally ill and mental health facilities in the local community. The deinstitutionalization of mental health care has meant that demands are placed on selected communities to act as host to a group which has traditionally been excluded by society in general. The reaction of the local community in its role as host is regarded as fundamental to the success of community-based care. Rejection of the mentally ill by local residents is likely to undermine any therapeutic benefit of being part of a 'normal' environment. As a result, an understanding of community response to the mentally ill and to the facilities which serve them is required for decisions about the planning and location of such facilities.

Faced with the possibility of having a mental health facility located in their neighbourhood, residents are typically sympathetic in principle toward the policy of treating the mentally ill in community rather than in institutional settings, but resistant in practice to a facility in the immediate neighbourhood. In this book we seek to determine whether this is an accurate description of public opinion. The questions we address include: Is the public in general sympathetic toward community-based mental health care? Does this sympathy turn to distrust and rejection because of the proposed location of a facility in a residential neighbourhood? What factors affect the degree of rejection? What negative impacts is the facility or are the clients expected to have? Are there groups within the general population who are more accepting of the mentally ill? Equally, are there particular types of neighbourhood which are more accepting? What implications do such social and spatial variations in public acceptance and rejection have for the location of facilities?

These are all relevant questions in the context of the policy of deinstitutionalization which has been widely adopted in North America, Britain, and elsewhere in the past twenty-five years. They are questions for which answers are largely lacking. The main reason for this is that until recently very little research has been devoted to them. The Toronto study, which forms the basis for much of this book, is one of the first attempts to undertake a comprehensive analysis of public attitudes toward the mentally ill in the community.

The approach we adopt is primarily geographical. We are ultimately concerned with identifying factors of importance for decisions about locating facilities in residential communities. At the same time, we recognize that this objective can only be achieved by a careful examination of the sociopsychological process which underlies community response to the mentally ill. Our theoretical model, which is based on recent work in attitude theory, reflects this conviction.

Although the substantive focus of the book is on the mentally ill and mental health facilities, the issues we address apply to a range of community-based services. The problems faced in the provision of facilities for the mentally ill are not unique to that group. We therefore regard our approach and results as having relevance for the analysis of public attitudes toward community-based services for other socially disadvantaged groups (for example, the mentally retarded, criminal offenders, drug offenders, and alcoholics).

This book should be of interest to several different groups whose professional background leads them to be concerned about public attitudes toward community health mental care and, more generally, toward social service provision. These groups include human geographers with interests in public facility location theory, a topic of growing concern in the discipline in recent years; social and community planners whose professional responsibilities include the provision of social services; and professionals in the mental health field. The book should also be of interest to sociologists and social and environmental psychologists given its focus on the process of attitude formation in the urban environment.

We are indebted to many people and various agencies for their help with this research. We gratefully acknowledge the financial support of the Canadian Social Sciences and Humanities Research Council. Two research grants supported the data collection and analysis, and leave fellowship awards to both authors facilitated completion of the book. Special thanks go to the group of graduate students who have worked with us—Brent Hall, John Boeckh, Bob Hughes, Steven Isaak, Kathie Jones, and Irene Wittman. Their contributions have frequently exceeded what was required to meet their own needs for thesis and dissertation completion. We are particularly grateful to Brent Hall for his help in editing and commenting on the final manuscript. The comments of Allen Scott, in his capacity as series editor, have also been very constructive and much appreciated. We are also indebted to Michael Poulson of Pion Ltd for his careful editing. We thank the staff of the Survey Research Centre at York University, Toronto, who had responsibility for the data collection for the Toronto attitude survey and compliment them on the quality and efficiency of their work. Thanks are also due to the following groups involved with mental health care in Metropolitan Toronto for providing information on the existing facilities and services in the Toronto area: Community Resources Consultants; the Canadian Mental Health Association; and personnel at Lakeshore Psychiatric Hospital, Queen Street Mental Health Centre, and the Clark Institute for Psychiatry. We also appreciate the cooperation of the Metropolitan Toronto Real Estate Board for allowing access to information on property transactions. Last, but not least, we are indebted to the 1090 residents of Toronto who participated in the questionnaire survey and to the additional people who responded to the pretest surveys.

Michael Dear, S Martin Taylor
Hamilton, Ontario, May 1982

Acknowledgements

We wish to thank the following organizations and journals for permission to reproduce copyright material:

The Association of American Geographers, Washington, DC, for figures 8.1, 8.2, and tables 7.1, 8.1–8.5;

The Canadian Association of Geographers, Montreal, for tables 9.1–9.8;

Regional Science Association, University of Illinois at Urbana–Champaign, for table 2.1;

Schizophrenia Bulletin, US Department of Health and Human Services, Public Health Service, Alcohol, Drug Abuse, and Mental Health Administration, Rockville, Maryland, for tables 6.1–6.3, 7.3–7.5, 7.8;

Social Science and Medicine, Pergamon Press, Oxford, for tables 7.9–7.11;

York University Geographic Monographs, Downsview, Ontario, for tables 2.2, 6.4.

To Heather and Avril

Contents

Contents

Part 1: Introduction

1 Content and context

The last twenty-five years has seen a major shift away from the use of large institutions for the treatment of the mentally ill. An increasing proportion of clients in need are now being treated in small-scale community-based facilities. These facilities vary considerably in their function, type, and size, but generally have in common their location in or close to residential neighbourhoods. The motives for a move away from institution-based treatment have been partly therapeutic, stemming from the social psychiatric view that the well-being of many patients is best served by their being part of a 'normal' environment, and partly economic, based on the desire to achieve reductions in the costs of providing care. Our concern, however, is not so much with the causes of deinstitutionalization as with its consequences for the community.

An immediate consequence of deinstitutionalization has been the demand placed on the community to act as host to a group which has traditionally been excluded by society in general. Indeed, as we later show, the concept of institutionalized care grew out of a desire to remove an unwanted group from everyday society to places where they could be effectively forgotten by the community at large. For the community willingly to accept the role of host to the mentally ill obviously therefore calls for a wholesale revision of conventional public attitudes. Survey data suggest that public attitudes have changed since World War 2, that there now exists a more open-minded and tolerant view of the mentally ill than at any time in the past. Indeed, there may be quite widespread acceptance in principle of the community mental health movement, but the critical question is whether such acceptance demonstrates itself in practice by a willingness to accept a mental health facility and its users in the same neighbourhood or even on the same street. There is sufficient evidence, much of it journalistic, to show that there is often considerable resistance from local residents to the location of a facility in their neighbourhood. Although the factors underlying such opposition are not well understood, it is clear that the shift to community-based mental health care has to take public attitudes into account.

Public attitudes to the mentally ill and to the facilities which serve them are of fundamental importance for the success of deinstitutionalized care in two ways. First, from the perspective of the ex-psychiatric patients, the attitudes of residents in neighbourhoods where facilities are located are of great importance in determining their social integration in the community. The potential therapeutic value of being part of a 'normal' environment can be seriously weakened or entirely lost if local residents demonstrate rejecting attitudes. In this regard, Rabkin (1977) observes that the increased contact between the mentally ill and the general public resulting from deinstitutionalization may engender friction in neighbourhoods, to the extent that "... if the force of public attitudes is not taken into account, the eventual outcome may be the exacerbation of public fears accompanied by a retreat to custodial care and removal from the community". Although this may be an overly pessimistic appraisal of possible future outcomes, it forcefully emphasizes the important implications that public attitudes toward the mentally ill have for the long-term development of community mental health care. The immediate question arising from Rabkin's assertion is in what ways should public attitudes be taken into account? The logical starting point would seem to be to establish the factors underlying these attitudes. What fears or uncertainties lead to individual and community opposition? Are these feelings limited to subgroups within the population or are they shared more widely? What could be done to generate positive and supportive views? There are many social and government agencies currently grappling with these kinds of questions, often on an ad hoc basis, seeking for practical solutions to the problem of locating a specific facility. Also emerging, however, are more systematic efforts by social researchers to investigate these same issues. Fundamental to these efforts is the desire to achieve a successful integration of the mentally ill into the community in the hope of promoting their return to 'normal' life-styles.

The second major reason why public attitudes toward the mentally ill are important relates to planning. Deinstitutionalization presents government and social service agencies with a very difficult task, namely to provide a network of facilities adequate to meet the needs of patients discharged from hospital and of those who would previously have been sent to hospital-based institutions. In many instances, the decrease in the number of institutionalized patients and the consequent increase in community care clients has been so rapid that the demand for community facilities has inevitably outreached the supply. The gap has been partially met, but there remains the need to establish many more purposely created facilities in the community. Public opposition to such facilities clearly accentuates an already difficult problem for local agencies. Different strategies have been tried to overcome the problem, ranging from siting a facility without prior consultation with local residents in the hope that a de facto location will effectively nullify potential opposition, to encouraging public involvement in the planning of a facility with the objective of educating them to the need to care for the mentally ill in the community, and with the desire to foster a positive and supportive neighbourhood environment. It is not clear at this point which strategy is ultimately the more successful. Although the open dialogue approach seems superficially to involve less risk of generating strong opposition, it certainly allows, and to some extent encourages, the expression of negative attitudes which may not necessarily lessen in the course of consultation. The basic point to recognize, however, is that regardless of the strategy adopted, the planner is considerably aided in any decision by a knowledge of the likely community response to proposed facility locations and of the factors affecting those responses.

Whether considered from the perspective of the client in need or the planner, public attitudes toward the mentally ill and toward community mental health facilities are of considerable importance. The desire to maximize the integration of the client in the community while minimizing the social and political conflict over facility locations calls for a careful analysis of the nature, extent, and underlying causes of public attitudes, and of the links between these attitudes and behavioural intentions and actions. To date there has been very little work in this area. Although attitudes toward mental illness and the mentally ill have long been studied, very little previous research has focussed on attitudes to the mentally ill in the community; much of the work has focussed on institutionalized care and predates the community mental health movement. Equally, the closely aligned issue of attitudes and reactions to facilities has until very recently received little or no attention. The research void is not surprising. As long as the mentally ill were removed from the community, studies of this sort were hardly relevant. However, the rapid advent of community-based care (in mental health and many other social services) makes such research not only relevant, but as we have implied, potentially vital.

The focus of this book is a response to this urgent need for a systematic investigation of public reaction to the mentally ill in the community. Our approach is inevitably coloured by our background as geographers. We are ultimately interested in the implications of public attitudes for locational decisions, but we recognize that these can only be worked out through the development and testing of a theoretical model which accurately describes the social and psychological processes underlying individual and community responses to the mentally ill and their facilities. With the substantive context for our work having been established, it is therefore appropriate that we next give a brief outline of its theoretical foundations.

1.1 Theoretical foundations
The substantive focus of this book, community attitudes to the mentally ill and to mental health facilities, is rooted in two main bodies of theory: public facility location theory and the theory of attitude formation.

Mental health facilities are one of many types of service which are normally provided by government through the expenditure of public funds. As such they are public facilities. Location theory as traditionally developed in economics, geography, and regional science focusses on locational decisions in the private sector. Recognition of the differences in locational decisionmaking in the public sector has resulted in the development of a distinctive public facility location theory. Perhaps the major distinguishing characteristic of this theory is the importance placed on the social and political process underlying locational decisions in the public sector. Efficiency-based models, typical of private sector theory, have been found inadequate, and equity considerations have been explicitly incorporated. The advent of equity criteria has meant that cost minimization in the supply of goods and services has had to be balanced against the social justice of locational decisions both for users and for nonusers.

Within public facility location theory, equity considerations require that locational decisions be viewed from several different perspectives. Location as access emphasizes the accessibility of facility locations for potential users. Location as externality recognizes that facilities have spillover effects, some of which, particularly for the nonusers, may be negative and generate opposition. The general social context of public facility location determines the interplay between social policy and spatial outcomes within which the politics of state intervention are particularly crucial. We consider these issues in some detail in chapter 2. Recognition of the spatial externalities associated with facility locations is especially important because they have a direct bearing on community attitudes. Perceived external effects, if negative, are potential generators of opposition. If positive or neutral, they are likely to lead to acceptance or at least indifference on the part of the host community.

Public facility location theory therefore leads to the explicit recognition of nonuser attitudes to facilities as a vital consideration in locational decisionmaking. The theory of attitude formation provides a framework within which the development of these attitudes can be analyzed. Attitude formation has long been an area of study in social psychology. There have been conflicting schools of thought about how attitudes are formed and change. Recently, however, there has been an effort to achieve a synthesis, in the form of the theory of reasoned action proposed by Ajzen and Fishbein (1980). Basic to this theory is the assumption that social behaviour is the product of a rational thought process. It is not normally the result of a random set of factors or forces. Ajzen and Fishbein posit a sequential process within which attitudes play a central and mediating role. Specifically, behaviour is the immediate consequence of an individual's behavioural intentions. These in turn link back to attitudes, which compose subjective evaluations of the behaviour in question, that is, the extent to which the individual is positively or negatively disposed toward carrying out the behaviour. The antecedants of attitudes are the individual's salient beliefs which may be personal or societal in their origin. The factors leading to beliefs comprise a whole range of what are termed external variables in the sense that they are external to the individual's mental processes. These include social and demographic status variables and various contextual factors, for example, the physical and social characteristics of the individual's neighbourhood.

As we show in chapter 2, the Fishbein–Ajzen model provides a very appropriate framework for analyzing attitudes and behaviour toward the mentally ill and mental health facilities. For our purposes, it is reasonable to assume that attitudes and actions are the product of a rational rather than a random process. This is not to imply that beliefs, attitudes, and behaviours toward the mentally ill are rational in the sense of necessarily being grounded in reality, but rather in the sense of being consciously generated. The components of the theory of reasoned action therefore form the basis for our theoretical model of individual response to community mental health care. We identify plausible sets of external variables and beliefs underlying attitudinal and behavioural responses to community mental health facilities. This model is the main framework for the empirical part of our research which focusses on public attitudes to mental health facilities in Metropolitan Toronto.

1.2 Empirical objectives
The theoretical foundations of our inquiry lead directly to three major empirical objectives:
1. to explain the attitudinal and behavioural responses of nonusers to neighbourhood mental health facilities;
2. to determine the nature and extent of the impacts of mental health facilities on residential neighbourhoods; and
3. to establish the planning and policy implications of individual and community responses to facilities.

The first objective derives from the importance of nonuser attitudes to facilities within public facility location theory. Our particular approach to the analysis of these attitudes is based on the theory of reasoned action as briefly outlined in the previous section. We have already argued for the importance of understanding nonuser responses to the mentally ill and the facilities which serve them. We maintain that the reactions of residents in host communities are fundamental to the success of community mental health care because of their potential effects on the patient's social integration and because of their implications for the selection of facility locations. Existing evidence on nonuser attitudes is largely speculative and anecdotal. Our first objective, therefore, is motivated by the need for much stronger empirical evidence on the nature, extent, and causes of nonuser reactions to neighbourhood mental health facilities.

The second objective is also linked to public facility location theory. The theory asserts that public facilities generate spatial externalities or spillover effects on the surrounding community. In the case of controversial public facilities, which would include those serving the mentally ill, these external effects are often perceived as detrimental in various ways to neighbourhood quality. These perceptions of negative impacts have a direct bearing on community acceptance or rejection of proposed or existing facilities. Here, again, existing evidence on the nature and spatial extent of these impacts is weak, and we feel it important that stronger evidence be obtained if community reactions to these facilities are to be understood and if sensible planning decisions are to be made.

Our third objective is an obvious outgrowth of the previous two. Although our research is partly motivated by a desire to contribute to the theoretical work which underlies it, we recognize that the substantive problem which we address has immediate practical significance. We are anxious, therefore, to distil from our empirical analyses the implications for planning decisions about facility locations. We realize that research of this kind rarely, if ever, produces final answers to the related planning issues, but we are concerned to do more than pay lip service to the planning implications of our work, particularly in the final section of the book.

The geographical setting for our research is Metropolitan Toronto. In the last ten years, community mental health care has become an increasingly salient political issue in the city as the demand for neighbourhood-based facilities has grown in response to the growing number of discharged hospital patients. A range of facilities has emerged providing both residential and nonresidential care services. Zoning restrictions and exclusionary policies by suburban boroughs have resulted in the concentration of facilities in a few city neighbourhoods, a phenomenon which has been described elsewhere as an 'asylum without walls'. The evolution of community mental health care in Toronto appears to be proceeding in similar ways to those observed in many other North American cities, even though the development of community-based care in Canada has proceeded more slowly than in the United States.

Reliance upon data from a single city inevitably raises questions about the generalizability of any findings. We cannot make strong assertions about the representativeness of Toronto as a North American city. At the same time, there are no obvious characteristics which make it clearly unique as a social research setting. We proceed, therefore, on the basis that Toronto provides a reliable and convenient laboratory for pursuing our research objectives, and we hope that those reading this book will find the results of our inquiry instructive and applicable to other urban areas.

1.3 Plan of the book
The book is divided into five parts: theoretical approach and study background; research design; individual response to neighbourhood mental health facilities; neighbourhood impacts of mental health facilities; and planning the location of mental health facilities.

The theoretical approach and study background comprises three chapters. In chapter 2, we discuss the theoretical basis for our analysis of community attitudes to mental health care. As indicated in the previous section, we draw upon two main bodies of theory: public facility location theory and the theory of attitude formation. In chapters 3 and 4 we examine two topics which are essential background to our inquiry. The first of these is the social history of the asylum, which presents a short historical overview of the treatment of the mentally ill from which we trace the origins of the community mental health movement. In chapter 4, we discuss previous research on attitudes toward the mentally ill. This literature provides important guidelines for our research, particularly to the extent that it identifies the types of beliefs which the public hold toward the mentally ill, the factors which influence these beliefs, and methods for measuring them.

The section on research design contains two chapters. The first (chapter 5) outlines the design of the Toronto study, specifically the data requirements, sample selection procedures, and questionnaire construction. The second (chapter 6) describes the development of two sets of belief scales which are important components in the subsequent empirical analysis. These scales measure beliefs about mental illness and neighbourhood beliefs.

The next section begins the empirical analysis and comprises a single chapter which presents the test of the theoretical model of individual response to neighbourhood mental health facilities developed in chapter 2. A sequence of relationships is tested by use of the Toronto data to determine the extent to which attitudes and behavioural intentions toward mental health facilities can be explained on the basis of an individual's beliefs and of a range of external variables.

The empirical analysis is continued in the next section which focusses on the neighbourhood impacts of mental health facilities. Neighbourhood impacts are examined in two ways. In chapter 8, the questionnaire survey data are used to examine the external effects which the public associate with mental health facilities. In chapter 9, real estate data for Metropolitan Toronto are used to test whether the introduction of facilities into residential neighbourhoods has had a measurable effect on property values. Property value decline is a commonly voiced fear and an especially prominent reason for opposing facility locations. Our analysis shows for Toronto whether this fear has any basis in fact.

The final section turns attention to the planning implications of our data and analysis. In chapter 10, we use the questionnaire data, together with census and land-use information, to develop profiles of neighbourhood acceptance and rejection of facilities. The prediction of the characteristics of accepting and rejecting neighbourhoods is then compared with the characteristics of the actual Toronto neighbourhoods where existing facilities are situated. This analysis is a first step toward the development of a planning tool which would enable planners to anticipate potential community response to proposed facility locations. In the final chapter, we summarize the main findings from our analyses and identify from them the policy implications of our work.

2 Analytical foundations: public facility location theory and the theory of attitude formation

This book concerns community attitudes toward the mentally ill and mental health facilities. The analytical foundations of this concern derive from two research areas: public facility location theory and the theory of attitude formation. The purpose of this chapter is to review the fundamental precepts of both these fields. The review is not meant to be exhaustive, since this would involve a detailed excursion into the diverse literatures of geography, psychology, regional science, sociology, and economics. Instead, we propose to review sufficient key materials to define a comprehensive theoretical model which will serve to guide the subsequent empirical analysis. Hence, in this chapter, the theory of public facility location and the theory of attitude formation are reviewed in the first two sections. Then, in the third section, our theoretical model is outlined.

2.1 Theory of public facility location

Public facilities are those units whose primary function is to deliver goods and services which fall wholly or partly within the domain of government. Such facilities have an important impact on urban form and environmental quality. The basis for a distinctive public facility location theory lies in the fact that decisions regarding such facilities are political decisions, involving public spending in response to a social welfare criterion in a mixed market/nonmarket setting. In contrast, a private sector location theory emphasizes individual choice, and utility-maximizing or profit-maximizing in a predominantly market context (Teitz, 1968, pages 37–38). As a consequence of the public dimension, any public facility location theory is not likely to be solely concerned with locational efficiency. Instead, such questions as the distributive impacts of the facility system and the influence of politics on public decisions will be of paramount importance.

2.1.1 The development of a distinctive theory of public facility location

The development of a distinctive contemporary theory of public facility location can be traced to Teitz's (1968) paper entitled "Toward a theory of urban public facility location". In this paper, the unique characteristics of the public sector problem were outlined, and an initial analytical framework was suggested. In the decade that followed, considerable literature developed around this theme. The power of Teitz's original formulation is attested by the fact that most of the subsequent research in this field has remained firmly within the boundaries established in this paper (see, for instance, the review by Hodgart, 1978). More recently, however, some far-reaching criticism of Teitz's approach has surfaced.

For instance, Dear (1978) argues for a fundamental realignment of public facility location theory because the strictures posed in the original paradigm are increasingly counterproductive. Even more fundamentally, Seley (1981a) has advocated a broadening of the approach to 'public services' analysis to incorporate a fuller consideration of the social welfare context of facility location. We shall return to these recent criticisms later in this section; we first trace the history which led up to them.

Analytical approaches to public facility location have varied. Teitz's attempts at alternative model formulations are indicative of many highly intractable problems. For instance, his simple static model is aimed at consumption-maximization of a zero-priced good supplied from a given spatial distribution of service facilities. Only the briefest sketch is given of a dynamic model (Teitz, 1968, pages 45–50). Perhaps the greatest single advance made by later researchers was to convert Teitz's micro-economic-based model into a more tractable mathematical programming framework. This allowed for a variety of improvements in modelling, including a more specific incorporation of the location variable, a wider range of social welfare surrogates as objective functions, and the addition of a hierarchical organization in the facility set (see the reviews by Freestone, 1977; and Lea, 1973).

Most of these public facility programming models have been derived from the private sector analogue. The typical private plant problem views location as a trade-off between facility and transport costs; hence, the greater the number of facilities, the lower the distribution costs, although this is only achieved by increased facility costs (ReVelle et al, 1970). This model has been converted to a public sector equivalent simply by substituting an objective function which represents 'social utility'. Characteristically, the problem of location in the public sector is expressed as designating m out of n sites as service locations, so as to minimize aggregate distance travelled by clients (ReVelle and Swain, 1970).

Several variations on this theme have been suggested. They reflect the search for a better specification of the reality of the public sector location process. For instance, the realization that 'accessibility' is only one aspect of social welfare has led to a search for a better surrogate in the objective function. Alternatives have included maximizing the demand created by the facility set, and minimizing the distance decay in utilization rates (Calvo and Marks, 1973). Other researchers have been content merely to tamper with the constraints of the model. Rojeski and ReVelle (1970), for example, replace the constraint of a fixed number of facilities by an upper limit on investment in facility costs.

The most recent contributions to this technical and methodological literature have reached a high level of sophistication. Notions of welfare are increasingly complex and have led to the development of multiobjective programming models (Bigman and ReVelle, 1978; 1979), and models which replicate the hierarchical organization typical of many public services.

For example, Dökmeci's multiobjective model for a four-tier regional
health system simultaneously aims to maximize utilization while
minimizing the sum of facility capital costs and user travel costs (Dökmeci,
1979). Others have attempted to introduce a greater realism into model-
building by incorporating behavioural constraints on consumer decisions.
For instance, Schuler and Holahan (1977) outline an optimizing framework
which emphasizes the effects of congestion on the size and spacing of
facilities. Also, Hodgson (1978), correctly assuming that consumers' travel
behaviour involves more than simply seeking out the closest facility, has
linked a location–allocation framework to an entropy-maximizing interaction model in order to allocate patrons to facilities.

In recognition of the political nature and redistributive consequences of
public facility location, other recent papers have begun to explore the
equity dimension of the location problem (Hodge and Gatrell, 1976;
Mumphrey and Wolpert, 1973). For instance, Wagner and Falkson (1975)
have suggested maximizing the sum of producers' and consumers' surpluses
for a given facility set, whereas McAllister (1976) has treated the equity-
efficiency trade-off in facility location. In McAllister's model, efficiency
is measured by the quantity of service demanded for a given budget; the
principal source of inequity is distance, as represented by the size and
spacing of centres. As might be anticipated, the equity and efficiency
goals are in conflict. Equity is high and efficiency low in a system of
closely spaced centres; and equity is low and efficiency high in a widely
spaced system. As McAllister indicates, there is no endogenous criterion
for assessing the trade-off between efficiency and equity in his model.

The introduction of an equity dimension in public facility location
theory seems to require that some exogenously derived equity or justice
criterion be entered into the optimizing framework. This is the reason
that many researchers are continuing to explore an heuristic approach to
public facility location. For example, McGrew and Monroe (1975) defined
pure-efficiency and pure-equity solutions for a locational problem, and
utilized a search procedure to improve system equity subject to an
efficiency constraint. In addition, Hillsman and Rushton (1976) have
devised an algorithm which allows decisionmakers to depart from a
globally optimum locational situation in order to use their local knowledge
and preferences to devise a 'better' local plan.

The need to consider elements of decisionmaking discretion in the
model has also stimulated specific studies of the nature of public decisionmaking. Thus, increasing attention is being directed toward the conflict
which arises when communities oppose the siting of controversial public
facilities as a consequence of the external effects of the facility (Dear,
1976; Wolpert et al, 1975). A clear statement on the need to incorporate
externality-induced compensation principles in locational analysis is
provided by the dynamic programming approach of Austin et al (1970).

This model minimizes the costs of a 'facility package' which includes the sum of the fixed costs of the facility set plus costs of modifying the facilities to offset community opposition. This latter group of costs refers to 'auxiliary facilities' which are designed to modify the external effects of a noxious public facility; for example, a barrier to insulate residents from expressway noise. The facility package approach is a significant variation on the traditional themes not only because it emphasizes a balance between efficiency and equity in public location decisions, but also because it recognizes the significance of externalities in the location process. It is important to observe that equity in location is thus composed of two elements: a direct impact which is related to the delivery of service to a client population (where traditional concerns of equity in access are of paramount importance); and an indirect impact which affects the wider, nonclient population through the externality fields of the facility set (where infringements of amenity rights cause community opposition).

Other researchers have felt obliged to abandon the highly formalized mathematical programming framework for more flexible evaluation methodologies. These typically examine the locational equity of a given spatial configuration of facilities; the problem of generating the facility set is ignored. For example, Schneider and Symons (1971) propose an 'access-opportunity index'. This is a statistic whose mean is interpreted as an efficiency criterion; standard deviation as a measure of equity; and population percentage below some minimum standard as a welfare criterion. Another ingenious statistical approach has been suggested by Morrill (1974), who summarizes four criteria for facility location. For a given nonhomogeneous population distribution, (1) location at the bivariate median is efficient, in that aggregate travel is minimized; (2) location at the bivariate mean is more equal, though less efficient, since it is weighted according to population density; (3) location at the point of maximum potential is efficient, since it assumes a distance-decay effect in consumption and ignores the fringes of the population; and (4) location at the population centroid is most equitable, since it minimizes the greatest distance travelled by any individual. Little effort has yet been made to build upon those simple but useful evaluation statistics. However, a potentially innovative approach was recently reported by Bach (1980), who devised nine criteria of accessibility and access opportunity for use in the traditional optimizing framework.

It is but a small step from these equity evaluation statistics to the more traditional plan evaluation methodologies. These include cost effectiveness, cost–benefit, goals achievement matrix, planning balance sheet, and PPBS techniques (see the reviews by Lichfield, 1970; and McAllister, 1980). To varying degrees, these methodologies offer potentially significant information which would assist public decisionmaking, including (1) information on the incidence of costs and benefits amongst impacted groups, (2) incorporation of monetary, numerical, and nonquantitative variables into the decision matrix, and (3) clarification of those criteria upon which the public choice has to be based (for example, a cost–benefit ratio). Unfortunately, these techniques are complex and imprecise. The measurement problem is especially problematic. Their potential remains high, however, and it is difficult to account for the lack of attention paid to them by researchers in public facility location theory.

2.1.2 A comprehensive theory of public facility location

The prominent departures from traditional efficiency-oriented concerns of locational theory represent attempts to incorporate the public aspect of location decisions more specifically into the analysis. At the core of a 'public' sector theory is the concept of a public good or service. In the absence of a clearly defined demand function for public goods, collective action by state agencies becomes necessary in response to the perceived needs of the populace. Otherwise, these goods are underprovided or are not produced at all (Steiner, 1970). The degree of intervention to provide public goods and services falls between the extremes of a completely spontaneous private process and a wholly controlled public process. It is, of course, unusual for any good to be produced at either extreme of the continuum. Different degrees of intervention may be anticipated (1) according to the degree of private market failure, and (2) according to decisions made in the political arena. As a consequence, the provision of public goods and public facilities can only be explained with reference to two distinct components: first, a substantive component, which is solely concerned with the 'technical' characteristics of demand and supply of a particular good or service; and, second, a procedural component, which emphasises the political and administrative procedures which govern decisions about the provision of the good or service.

Although Teitz and others have been aware of the political (that is, procedural) aspects of public decisions, their analytical formulations have almost entirely focussed upon the substantive aspects of the location problem (compare Hodgart, 1978). Yet the procedural/substantive dichotomy is unsupportable, since the nature of public intervention cannot logically be separated from the socioeconomic and political context within which it is embedded. Procedural and substantive aspects inevitably act as mutual constraints. Hence, any public facility location theory must also be a theory of society, and it can only be understood as a manifestation of a given social order.

The point of view which regards public facility location theory as part of a wider social theory is implicit in many recent reviews of location theory. Wood (1977; 1978; 1979) has consistently advocated fuller attention to the 'institutional framework' of spatial behaviour, especially the 'manipulative ambitions' of bureaucracies. A more explicit advocacy of the social-theory approach is contained in a collection of papers edited by Seley (1981b). In adopting a wider definition of 'public services', Seley and his colleagues open up new horizons in this field. In his own contribution, Seley (1981c) explores the crucial social service needs of small businesses in metropolitan areas, whereas Reiner and Wolpert (1981) examine the links between the philanthropic behaviour of the nonprofit sector and metropolitan growth and decline (see also Wolpert, 1977). In addition, Wolch (1981) provides valuable insight into the characteristics of the service-dependent populations, emphasizing that their budgetary constraints are dominated by housing costs and transportation-to-service costs, and that facilities to serve them locate to minimize client transport costs. As a consequence, the service-dependent populations and their facilities congregate in poverty-ridden central city neighbourhoods. Such 'ghettoization' is a complex outcome of a wide range of social, political, and economic factors (Massey, 1980; Wolch, 1980; Wolpert, 1980).

On the basis of previous work (Dear, 1978), it is our view that a comprehensive public facility location theory should, first, be self-consciously embedded within a wider theory of society, in order that the forward and backward linkages may be clarified among the social formation, its concomitant public policy, and the spatial outcomes of that policy. Second, spatial outcomes, which form the focus of analysis, should be disaggregated into two components: the direct (anticipated) outcomes of the policy decision; and the indirect (unanticipated, externality-induced) outcomes. Both the direct and indirect outcomes of public decisions are a major source of variation in environmental quality and social well-being. The substantive impact of these outcomes is, therefore, an important source of procedural (that is, political) debate in the public decision process. Any comprehensive theory of public facility location should seek to explain spatial outcomes in terms of the dual (direct and indirect) impact of public decisions on social welfare, and to situate the public decisionmaking process within the wider social formation. Three analytical components are therefore essential in such a theory: (1) location as access, (2) location as externality, and (3) locational decisions in the context of the wider social formation. We briefly outline the significance of each of these factors, with special reference to the mental health care example.

Location as access

The influence of location on the utilization of public facilities has been widely conceded, although its specific role remains ambiguous. In the case of psychiatric care, for instance, Weiss et al (1966) have shown that the further patients reside from a mental hospital the more rigorous the diagnostic criteria which doctors exercise before discharging them. On the other hand, Smith (1976a) emphasizes the 'miniscule' effect of distance upon a patient's ability to stay out of hospital once discharged. Whatever the exact significance, it is important to emphasize that access to public

facility services is vital to the potential consumer. The availability of
a service may literally mean the difference between life and death.
Consequently, a dual hypothesis seems necessary for the analysis of public
facility utilization (Dear, 1978): (1) that location has little measurable
impact on the overall utilization of social services by the population at
risk (that is, the decision to seek care), and (2) that location has a
significant effect on a user's choice of a particular facility.

Support for this construct has been forthcoming from the many
continuing investigations into the role of accessibility in the utilization of
health services (for example, Joseph, 1979; Knox, 1978; Phillips, 1979;
and Stimson, 1980). However, White (1979) has commented that
accessibility is an inadequate criterion for public facility location, since it
places an overemphasis on facility dispersion as a locational solution. In
his 'colocational' analysis, he emphasizes the interaction and linkage
between similar facilities. Such agglomeration economies provide a potent
force for facility concentration (see below).

Previous research has suggested that three groups of characteristics
influence the utilization of mental health services: the characteristics of the
service being provided, the characteristics of the client population, and
the location of the service. The utilization decision of any consumer is
viewed as a function of fifteen variables (table 2.1). Different consumer
responses represent differential weightings on some or all of the fifteen
characteristics. It is unlikely that all variables will be relevant at all times.
More commonly, the variables will enter and leave the individual's decision
calculus with differential weights attached, according to specific situations.

Table 2.1. Variables influencing utilization of mental health care facilities (source:
Dear, 1978, page 102).

(A) *Service characteristics*	(B) *Client characteristics*
1 Intake policy, including facility opening times	7 Demographic factors
2 Quality and type of service	8 Income
3 Physical amenity of the service facility	9 Education
4 Size of facility	10 Religion
5 Capacity of facility	11 Presenting symptoms
6 Price of service	(C) *Location characteristics*
	12 Physical distance (accessibility)
	13 Location as catchment[a]
	14 Social distance[b]
	15 Relative location[c]

[a] In which rules governing the administrative area where clients may obtain service may
force the clients to ignore more accessible service alternatives.
[b] The 'distance' placed between client and service by referral patterns.
[c] The set of intervening service opportunities and why they may be ignored or accepted.

Location as externality

The primary emphasis on delivering a service to the consumer, or on making services accessible to consumers, obscures the important range of external effects generated by the location variable, as exemplified by White's work. Such externalities may affect both consumers (users) and nonconsumers (nonusers) of the facility's services. The former group may be designated as user-associated externalities, the latter group as neighbourhood-associated externalities.

The set of user-associated external effects is related to the concept of agglomeration economies. Although traditional emphasis on accessibility encourages a dispersed facility pattern, agglomerative criteria might warrant a concentrated pattern. The consumer will obviously benefit if all internal scale economies have been captured in a facility's operation. But, more significantly, urbanization and localization economies might encourage clustering of service facilities, such that users might be able to take advantage of choice, or make multiple-purpose visits (Wolch, 1980; White, 1979).

It is vital to note that although user attitudes toward service facility clusters are usually positive, nonuser attitudes are almost universally negative. The same facility set generates external effects which are perceived differently as neighbourhood-associated externalities by the 'host' community. Residents often appear to be concerned with the possible saturation of service facilities in their neighbourhood. A 'tipping' effect has already occurred in some cities, transforming what was once an area of residential land use into one of predominantly institutional uses.

From our viewpoint, interest in neighbourhood-associated externalities lies in the impetus it provides for locational conflict over facility siting. This is predominantly a procedural question which derives from the implementation costs associated with a particular service plan. Conflict studies have repeatedly emphasized the importance of facility externalities in community acceptance or rejection of a mental health program. Even apparently reasonable substantive plans for service delivery have been upset because the procedural problems associated with implementation have been ignored. Frequently, the opportunity to locate anywhere within a particular neighbourhood is denied, thereby causing a serious distortion in the pattern of service delivery.

Locational conflict over public facility location is usually based upon the perceived negative external effects of a facility, its users, or a multiple-facility complex. Two groups of external effects have been noticed: tangible effects, which are based upon clearly recognizable, usually quantifiable, impacts of the facility in question; and intangible effects, which refer to a wide range of nonquantitative impacts. The former group includes property value decline and increased traffic in the vicinity of the facility. The latter group includes fear for personal security, the stigma of mental illness, and dislike of loitering clients (Dear, 1976). A wide range of contextual variables also influences community response (see chapter 4; and Smith and Hanham, 1981).

In response to extensive community opposition to substantive plans for mental health facility siting, planners have developed numerous procedural strategies to avoid conflict. One of two approaches tends to be adopted: the 'low-profile' approach, which educates and coerces the community into accepting a facility before it is introduced; or the 'fly-by-night' strategy, which involves setting up a facility secretly, and hoping that it will not be noticed until its operation can demonstrably be shown to be harmless (Wolpert et al, 1975). However, since both strategies are hazardous, a third 'risk-aversion' strategy has become common. This involves seeking out locations where no community opposition is anticipated or where controversial facilities would go unnoticed. Such locations tend to proliferate in transient, rental accommodation areas of inner cities, thus accentuating the ghettoization trend noted in the previous section. As well as making location/siting concessions toward potentially opposing community groups, planners have also made financial concessions to impacted communities and have altered facility design to cope with specific objections.

The social context of public facility location
The two dimensions of location (as access and as externality) have produced two entirely different treatment settings in the case of mental health care. The first, based on access, has resulted in a decentralized system of community mental health facilities. The second, a consequence of aggregate external effects, has led to the organic creation of a ghetto of the mentally disabled. To assess the future of these two important service modalities, it is essential to place mental health in its proper policy context. For example, the ghetto is already being dismantled by zoning ordinances in a number of North American cities; this is in pragmatic response to community opposition to such ghettos, irrespective of their potentially positive service impact (Wolpert and Wolpert, 1976). To proceed with this analysis, it must be conceded that the pattern of provision is inextricably linked to the contemporary socioeconomic and political setting. Spatial outcomes must therefore seek their explanations in the wider social context; there is a direct correlation between social policy and spatial outcome. This link has tended to be ignored in favour of the technical problems inspired by the existing public facility location paradigm.

A social-context view of mental health care has several important consequences. First, mental health care is not only a technical problem of matching supply and demand. The actual service outcome is a consequence of the interaction among four groups which impinge upon the technical problem of service delivery. These groups are: the client in need, the professional care-giver, the community, and the state. The provision or nonprovision of care depends upon the demands of each group and upon the relative power of each group to achieve its demands (Dear, 1981). Second, with respect to the community, primary attention is focussed upon its role in accepting or rejecting the ex-psychiatric patient. As we suggested in chapter 1, neighbourhood acceptance of the mentally ill and mental health facilities is vital to the success of community-based care (Segal and Aviram, 1978; Smith and Hanham, 1981). This theory is taken up in detail again in chapter 4. Third, we are also concerned, but to a lesser extent, with the role of the state in the formation and implementation of mental health policy [for instance, through the practice of zoning and control of land use, compare Schmedemann (1979)]. Increasing attention is now being paid to the impact of state intervention on sociospatial outcomes (see reviews by Clark and Dear, 1978; Jessop, 1977; and Johnston, 1980; amongst others). We cannot hope to review this complex literature here. Instead, we are content merely to assert that a full appreciation of the themes of this book is possible only by recognizing the impact of the state on the social and spatial process which we are describing. The historical review of mental health care policy presented in chapter 3 is intended to provide (however briefly) the background necessary for this appreciation. Finally, our social-context viewpoint underlines the need to maintain a careful balance between the more aggregate (macroscale) factors governing social attitudes and spatial change and the individual behavioural (microscale) factors influencing specific sociospatial outcomes. We seek to incorporate both sets of factors in our theoretical model and analytical procedures.

2.1.3 Summary

Classical microeconomic and mathematical programming models have tended to dominate public facility location theory. More recently, however, awareness of the political nature of public facility location has directed attention toward the social welfare dimension of the location problem. Three main analytical approaches can be distinguished: location as access, location as externality, and the social context of public facility location. The last two, and especially location as externality, are relevant to our problem of determining community response to neighbourhood mental health facilities. This is because the mentally ill person and the mental health facility are sources of external effects in the location process. These externalities are fundamental in shaping community attitudes to facilities and thereby affect the integration of client and facility into a community. Our emphasis on community attitudes to facilities therefore reflects recent developments in public facility location theory. In short, we are concerned with understanding the nonuser aspect of the externality dimension, recognizing the vital importance that this can have in the successful location of controversial public facilities and specifically mental health facilities.

2.2 Community attitudes to public facilities

In the previous section we have set our work in the context of public facility location theory. We now consider within this general framework the particular approach that we have chosen to adopt in studying community response to neighbourhood mental health facilities—a case of location as externality. Our approach places central importance on the attitudes of residents in host communities for predicting and explaining the behavioural outcomes of primary concern, namely the acceptance or rejection of facilities. As a necessary prelude to formalizing our approach in a theoretical model, we address three issues in this section: the role of attitudes, the formation of attitudes, and the link between attitudes and behaviour.

2.2.1 The role of community attitudes

Our objective is to predict and explain community acceptance or rejection of neighbourhood mental health facilities. The degree of acceptance or rejection is the outcome of concern. We maintain that the prediction and explanation of a particular outcome depends upon understanding the attitudes of community residents toward a facility. We find support for this assertion in recent research on attitude theory and particularly the work of Fishbein and Ajzen (Fishbein and Ajzen, 1975; Ajzen and Fishbein, 1980). They have developed a theoretical framework for analyzing social behaviour. Within this framework, attitudes play a central role linking prior beliefs to specific behaviours. The details of the Fishbein–Ajzen model and its relevance to our specific research problem are best understood by way of an example.

Let us assume that a local planning authority has proposed to locate a group home for ex-psychiatric patients in the hypothetical neighbourhood of Hillside. News of this proposal has reached Hillside residents through reports in the local newspaper. Concern about the proposal has grown as groups of individuals within the neighbourhood have speculated about the impacts of the facility. This concern has culminated in the formation of a local action group which has demanded a meeting with the planning authority, where they can express their views and receive more details about the proposed facility. At the meeting a planner outlines the philosophy behind community mental health care and emphasizes the advantages to the patient from living within a 'normal' residential environment. Some Hillside residents in the audience become increasingly agitated as this presentation continues and mumbled comments gradually give way to deliberate interruptions. When the planner has finished, a particularly vociferous resident gets up and makes it clear that, although he has some sympathy for the problems faced by ex-psychiatric patients, he does not see why he and his neighbours should have to bear the responsibility and risks which hosting the facility could engender. He expresses fears about the potential danger posed by the facility to all members of the community and particularly to the children. He worries about a detrimental effect on property values and the possibility that allowing the location of one facility would be opening the door to several more. As he continues it is obvious that he is increasingly winning the support of his fellow residents at the meeting. Attempts by the planning officials to give reassurance about the composition and running of the home have little effect and the meeting ends with a near unanimous rejection of the proposal by the residents. The planning officials leave wondering whether the group home is a feasible venture given the level of opposition that has been expressed.

From this simplified but not untypical scenario, we note first that the outcome was community rejection of the facility. What factors led to this outcome? Quite obviously, it was an immediate consequence of the behaviour of particular individuals within the intended host community. The specific behaviours undertaken include the formation of an action group, attendance at the community meeting, and vocal expression of views during the meeting. It is reasonable to suppose that these behaviours were not randomly generated, but rather the product of conscious intentions on the part of the individuals involved. The opposition observed is a consequence of deliberate behavioural intentions. The formation of an action group was preceded by definite intentions among community members to form such a group. Equally, those in attendance at the meeting had intended to be there, and those who expressed their feelings had intended to do so.

The question that logically follows concerns the origins of these intentions. Again, if we are prepared to assume that the types of observed behaviour are the product of a rational process, it is reasonable to suppose that behavioural intentions arise out of a conscious evaluation of the value of undertaking each specific behaviour. In simple terms, this implies that the individuals (either independently or jointly) evaluated the value of forming an action group, attending the meeting, speaking out, and so on. In essence, this evaluation process involves the formation of attitudes toward the behaviour in question. To this point, therefore, our analysis of the factors leading to the observed outcome of community rejection of the proposed facility has identified a *sequential process* whereby attitudes toward particular behaviours give rise to behavioural intentions, which are the immediate antecedents of the behaviours themselves, which in turn lead directly to the outcome (rejection).

The factors underlying attitudes toward behaviour must be understood if an explanation of outcomes is to be achieved. Essentially, this involves identifying salient beliefs. Returning to the scenario we can discern some clues about the nature of these factors. The spokesman for the community expressed various fears about the possible detrimental impacts of the proposed group home. These fears constitute personal beliefs about the potential effects of the facility location. Such beliefs have a direct bearing on the formation of attitudes. For example, believing that allowing the facility into the neighbourhood may endanger the safety of children leads to the belief that opposing the facility will have a desirable outcome, namely preventing the source of potential danger. This latter belief leads directly to the formulation of an attitude toward oppositional behaviour. For example, attendance at a protest meeting may be evaluated as a good thing because it can contribute toward achieving the desired outcome. Notice, however, that within the scenario the *salient beliefs* are not necessarily consistent with each other. The spokesman for the community admitted some sympathy for the needs of ex-psychiatric patients, implying that in principle he could accept the philosophy of community mental health care as previously expounded by the planner. This suggests that the formation of attitudes toward behaviour may involve a balancing of conflicting beliefs, which implies assigning weights to them to determine the degree of influence each should have on attitudes. In the scenario, beliefs about the detrimental effects of a group home outweighed beliefs about the positive benefits such a facility could provide to ex-psychiatric patients, and led to an attitude favouring oppositional behaviour.

Notice also that we can distinguish between these beliefs in terms of those which are normative and those which are not. *Normative beliefs* are those which an individual holds because others whom he respects and wants to conform with expound them. In some cases these beliefs may be very generally accepted within a society (for example, the belief that it is wrong to commit murder); in other cases, they may be more limited in their acceptance, as in our illustration with the belief about the merit of community mental health care. Acceptance by the community spokesman of the positive benefit for ex-psychiatric patients of a group home represented a normative belief.

We have now added beliefs to the set of factors underlying the outcome which we are concerned to explain. The sequence to this point therefore involves *beliefs* leading to *attitudes*, leading to *behavioural intentions*, leading to *behaviour*, leading to *outcomes*. This reductionist approach can be taken a stage further to identify the *factors giving rise to beliefs*. Here we may be concerned with a variety of personal and situational variables, which exert an external influence on the psychological process described up to this point. Important personal variables include demographic characteristics. We might expect residents with young children, for example, to have different beliefs about the consequences of the group home than those without. Economic status might be important, home owners perhaps holding different beliefs from those who rent their homes. Personality traits might also be influential, as, for example, in the extent to which individuals are authoritarian or aggressive. In terms of situational variables, neighbourhood and facility characteristics would seem to be important. We would anticipate beliefs to vary in relation to the size of the proposed facility, for example, and also with respect to the characteristics of the intended residents. Beliefs might also be expected to differ dependent upon the mixture of commercial, institutional, and residential properties in the host neighbourhood, since these factors may affect the visibility of the facility. To identify the antecedents of beliefs, therefore, involves dealing with a complex of variables, the effects of any one of which is often very difficult to isolate.

Based on our simple scenario we have traced the process leading to the outcome of community rejection (or acceptance) of a facility. Within this process, attitudes toward behaviour play a central and mediating role linking salient beliefs with behavioural intentions and behaviour. This conceptualization of the process underlying social behaviour and of the role of attitudes within it follows the theory of reasoned action proposed by Fishbein and Ajzen (1975). They conceive of a sequential process involving beliefs, attitudes, behavioural intentions and behaviour. They also recognize that many 'external variables' (for example, demographic, social, and personality factors) influence this process particularly through their effects on the formation of beliefs. They are careful to distinguish between normative and nonnormative beliefs and regard the relative weighting of these as basic to attitude formation and behavioural intentions. Fishbein and Ajzen stress that success in predicting behaviour from attitudes or attitudes from beliefs requires that the objects to which each component refers correspond. They argue that lack of correspondence accounts in large measure for the failure in previous studies to show strong relationships between attitudes and behaviour.

2.2.2 The formation of community attitudes
In the previous section, attitudes were defined as positive or negative evaluations of behaviours perceived to lead to particular outcomes. It follows that an individual should hold a positive attitude toward a behaviour perceived to lead to a desired outcome and a negative attitude toward behaviours leading to undesired outcomes. It is important to notice that we are here referring to *attitudes toward behaviour* rather than *attitudes toward particular objects* which may be the referents for the behaviour. Following the Fishbein–Ajzen theory of reasoned action, attitudes toward salient objects (for example, mental health facilities and the mentally ill) fall into the category of behavioural or normative beliefs. As such, they correspond to the cognitive rather than evaluative component of attitudes. We need to identify salient beliefs if we are to explain the formation of attitudes toward facility acceptance or rejection.

Ajzen and Fishbein (1980) argue that, with respect to a particular social behaviour, an individual holds two types of belief. These are *behavioural beliefs* which are generated from personal perceptions of the consequences of the behaviour, and *normative beliefs* which are a function of social influences which have a bearing on the behaviour. Certain individuals might believe that by opposing the opening of a mental health facility a fall in neighbourhood property values is likely to be prevented. This would constitute a behavioural belief. They might also believe that, by accepting the facility, they are fulfilling what those in authority regard as their responsibility to do the best they can for humanity. This would be a normative belief since it is primarily a response to the expectations of others.

For present purposes, therefore, our task is to identify the behavioural and normative beliefs connected with facility acceptance or rejection. These beliefs focus upon three elements: the facility, the users of the facility, and the neighbourhood. We have already hinted that the salient beliefs regarding the facility might entail beliefs about the possible impacts of the facility on the neighbourhood and on the local residents. The impacts could include personal safety, property value effects, and future facility saturation, as well as traffic volumes, noise levels, aberrant behaviour, and neighbourhood character. Previous research provides some direction for identifying relevant impacts (Dear et al, 1977) as do reports in the media about neighbourhood opposition to facilities (see table 2.2). With respect to each impact, beliefs are potentially positive (for example, the location of a facility in my neighbourhood will increase property values), negative (the facility location will decrease property values), or neutral (the facility will have no effect on property values).

Beliefs about the users of facilities, the mentally ill, have been the subject of extensive research (for reviews see Rabkin, 1972; 1974; and 1975) which is discussed in detail in chapter 4. This work has led to the identification of different psychological dimensions on which public beliefs about the mentally ill are based, and the development of standardized scaling instruments to measure each dimension. The most widely applied scales are the 'opinions about mental illness' scales developed by Cohen and Struening (1962) which distinguish five separate dimensions: authoritarianism, benevolence, social restrictiveness, mental hygiene ideology, and interpersonal etiology. Also important, particularly with

Table 2.2. Bases for resident oppositions to community mental health facilities—recorded at least once in *The Toronto Globe and Mail* or *The Toronto Star*, January 1977 to May 1978. (Source: Isaak et al, 1980, page 235.)

Increase in noise	Illegal operation
Decrease in property sale	Nonprofessional care
Increase in traffic	Lack of supervision
Increase in parking problems	Dislike of facility users
Poorly run homes in respectable neighbourhoods	Fear for personal or family safety: fear of arson
Building not maintained	fear of theft
Detract from neighbourhood quality	fear of vandalism
Detract from neighbourhood stability	fear of assault
Poor administration	fear of rape
	fear of murder

reference to community mental health care, is the community mental health ideology scale (CHMI) developed by Baker and Schulberg (1967). Although these scales are commonly referred to as attitude scales, they essentially measure the belief component of attitudes and so are more appropriately regarded as belief measures in the context of the Fishbein–Ajzen model.

Beliefs about the neighbourhood are perhaps less easily identified. Intuitively, they are based on perceptions of the suitability of the neighbourhood as a host for a mental health facility. This may be disaggregated into perceptions of the physical and social characteristics of the neighbourhood and the extent to which each are congruent with the proposed facility. The concept of congruence is inherently intangible and yet potentially very important for understanding community response to facilities. It corresponds to the notion of 'fit' between form and context as articulated in the architectural and design literature (Alexander, 1964). To illustrate, we could expect residents in a completely residential suburban development to perceive their neighbourhood as unsuited for the location of a store-front, drop-in centre for ex-psychiatric patients, since such a facility would be incongruent with existing land uses. Equally, we can conceive of beliefs about the suitability of the neighbourhood based on the perceived congruence between the characteristics of local residents and of the proposed users of the facility. A facility designed primarily to serve the needs of local residents might well be perceived as more congruent and, hence, more suitable than one established to serve outsiders.

In analysing the formation of attitudes we may look beyond the beliefs which immediately antecede them and attempt to identify the external variables which are correlated with beliefs. We may wish to do this to increase the explanatory power of our analysis (to document more completely why certain outcomes occur). Studies which focus on external variables as the basic explanatory factors are common in behavioural research. However, in large measure, they have achieved disappointing results. The relationships reported between external variables (such as demographic, social, and personality characteristics) and various social behaviours have generally been weak.

The usefulness of external variables in a particular study depends very much on the research objectives. If the major aim is to achieve accurate predictions of behaviour, it is unlikely that external variables will be of much value. On the other hand, if the primary concern is to uncover the factors underlying behaviour, such variables may be extremely valuable. A reasonable criticism of the Fishbein–Ajzen theory is that it is relatively arid as an explanatory framework, because the determinants of behaviour which it incorporates are so close to the behaviour as to be redundant in explaining it. This applies especially to behavioural intentions, the immediate antecedents of behaviour, but also seems to apply to beliefs even though to a lesser extent. For this reason, we place greater emphasis on the role of external variables than do Fishbein and Ajzen in their theory of reasoned action. To downplay the importance of external variables has the danger of reducing the explanatory power of the theory to an epiphenomenal level. We immediately recognize the important influence of a range of environmental, social, and personal factors on responses to community mental health facilities and incorporate these within our theoretical framework as the antecedants of beliefs, attitudes, and intentions.

2.2.3 Community attitudes and behaviour

The relationship between attitudes and behaviour has been an issue of major controversy in the attitude literature dating back to LaPiere's classic study (LaPiere, 1934). To some extent attitude theorists have been able to avoid the issue by concentrating on the dynamics of attitude formation without reference to the links to behaviour. However, the catalogue of empirical studies involving attitude–behaviour relationships raises serious questions. Wicker's review of these studies succinctly states the problem: "It is considerably more likely that attitudes will be unrelated or only slightly related to overt behaviours than that attitudes will be closely related to actions" (Wicker, 1969, page 65). Must we, therefore, conclude that attitudes are in principle useful, but in practice useless, variables for behavioural analysis? More recent work suggests not.

Fishbein and Ajzen (1975) show that many of the empirical studies included in Wicker's review fail to demonstrate strong relationships between measures of attitude and behaviour because of a lack of correspondence in the measurements used. Attitudes were typically measured with reference to general objects or targets whereas behaviour was measured in terms of specific actions. In the mental health context, an example could be that of relating measures of an employer's attitudes toward the mentally ill to willingness to hire discharged psychiatric patients. Fishbein and Ajzen contend that at best only a weak relationship could be expected, because the attitude being measured does not correspond to the behaviour in question. The appropriate attitude to measure in this case would be the employer's attitude toward hiring ex-psychiatric patients. In Ajzen and Fishbein's words the guiding principle is that "... to predict a single behaviour we have to assess the person's attitude toward the target at which the behaviour is directed" (Ajzen and Fishbein, 1980, page 27). Notice, this does not rule out the possible usefulness of general attitudes toward objects for predicting an overall pattern of behaviour. Since overall patterns of behaviour may well be our concern in community mental health studies, we would be wrong to dismiss general measures of attitudes as being unfruitful. Also, as previously indicated, we are often more concerned with the behaviour of aggregates rather than of single individuals, and here, again, general measures of attitudes (averaged over a group) can be expected to show stronger relationships than the same general measures used in a disaggregate analysis.

The net conclusion seems to be that, by paying due attention to the guidelines provided in the most recent literature, attitude measures can be successfully employed for studying behaviour, and that this is especially true where the focus is on overall behavioural patterns and aggregate behaviour rather than on the prediction of individual actions. For these reasons, we conclude that making community attitudes the basis for studying facility acceptance and rejection is valid despite the doubts expressed in previous research about the attitude–behaviour relationship.

2.2.4 Summary
Community attitudes are basic to an understanding of community response to neighbourhood mental health facilities. Consistent with current attitude theory, attitudes are conceived as a central component within a sequential process linking beliefs to behavioural outcomes. The explanation and prediction of attitudes therefore depends upon the identification and measurement of salient sets of beliefs. To further the explanatory power and practical utility of any analysis, it is also necessary to examine the factors influencing belief formation which include a variety of personal and situational variables. The issue of the relationship between attitudes and behaviour was examined. In light of recent attitude research, the weak relationship shown in earlier studies is not considered a reason for rejecting an attitudinal approach for the analysis of community response to mental health facilities.

2.3 The theoretical model
The theoretical model for our study of community response to neighbourhood mental health facilities is developed from the recent work in attitude theory discussed in the previous section. In particular Fishbein and Ajzen's theory of reasoned action provides the basic structure for the model. The model has six major components: external variables, beliefs, attitudes, behavioural intentions, behaviour, and outcomes (figure 2.1). The first two of these break down into a number of subcomponents.

2.3.1 External variables
Three separate sets of external variables affect the formation of salient beliefs. These are facility characteristics, neighbourhood characteristics, and personal characteristics. The first two are situational or contextual attributes which are defined at a neighbourhood scale and the last are measured at the individual level. Individual beliefs, attitudes, intentions, and behaviour are therefore regarded as the product of an interaction of variables at two levels, the individual and the aggregate (where the latter corresponds to the individual's neighbourhood). The first set of external variables comprises the characteristics of the facility and of the facility users. Both are linked directly to beliefs about facility impacts. Important facility characteristics include its size, design, level of supervision, and the type of service offered. The last would seem especially important.

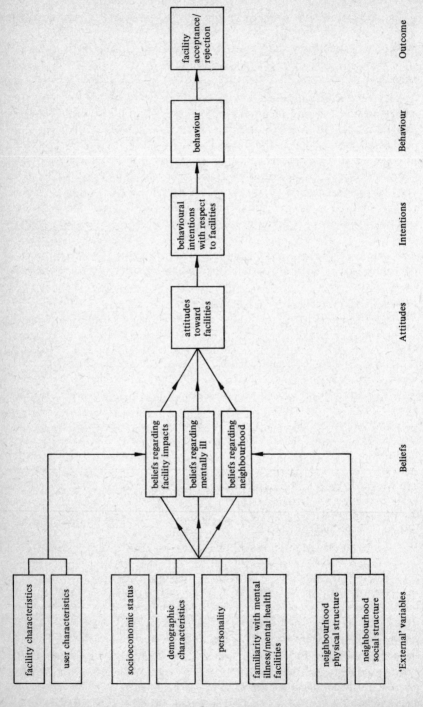

Figure 2.1. Theoretical model of community attitudes to mental health care.

It is vital to recognize the variety of service types embraced by the label
'community mental health facility'. The term includes residential care
facilities, which encompass a range spanning from commercial boarding
homes to organized group homes, outpatient services, social and therapeutic
programs, and vocational services. We might expect community residents
to have very different beliefs about the potential impacts of residential
and nonresidential care facilities, for example. The former brings the ex-
psychiatric patient into the neighbourhood on a permanent or semipermanent basis, whereas the latter involves only brief visits by clients.
In principle we would anticipate that the larger the facility the greater its
potential impact. With regard to design, the visibility of the facility is
particularly significant. A facility which has the same external appearance
as neighbouring properties is likely to have a lesser impact than one which
is very conspicuous. This hypothesis is consistent with the concept of fit
between form and context. Type and level of supervision are likely to
influence the beliefs of local residents about the impact of the facility on
personal safety. A facility which is continuously supervised by professional
staff will probably be viewed as less of a threat than one which is only
partially supervised or totally unsupervised.

User or client characteristics cannot be entirely divorced from the type
of facility, although any one facility may serve the needs of various
groups. The literature on attitudes toward the mentally ill provides some
basis for inferring which client characteristics might affect beliefs about
facility impacts. For instance, the sex and socioeconomic status of
patients have been shown to influence the degree of rejection of the
mentally ill (Linsky, 1970; Phillips, 1964). Males and those of lower
economic status were found to be more often and more strongly rejected.
More vital, however, are the visibility of deviant behaviour and the extent
to which it is perceived as unpredictable and dangerous. Bizarre and
disruptive behaviour is rejected more strongly than withdrawal (Lemkau
and Crocetti, 1962). Unpredictability and dangerousness have invariably
been associated with strong rejection (Bord, 1971). Not surprisingly it is
the outward appearances more than the underlying symptomatology that
influence public beliefs and fears about facility users.

The second set of external variables comprises personal characteristics
which divide into four subsets. Each subset has a potential influence on
each of the three sets of salient beliefs. The first subset consists of
socioeconomic status variables, namely income, education, and occupation.
Income, for example, might influence beliefs about facility impacts
through its relationship with home ownership and hence with fears about
the property value effects of facilities. Education is likely to affect
knowledge about mental illness and thereby beliefs about the mentally ill.
Occupational status affects neighbourhood beliefs (Michelson, 1970) and
particularly beliefs about suitable types of neighbours. Demographic
characteristics comprise the second subset of personal characteristics.

Life-cycle stage is probably the most important factor in this category because the presence and ages of children in the household has an important influence on all three sets of beliefs. Beliefs about the personal danger posed by a facility and its users are an obvious example. Personality characteristics make up the third subset. Their influence is perhaps less easily anticipated. One frequently measured personality dimension, authoritarianism, seems particularly relevant and this is confirmed by the fact that Cohen and Struening (1962) apply that label to one of the dimensions they identify in their scaling of opinions about the mentally ill. The fourth and final subset of personal characteristics is familiarity with the mentally ill and mental health facilities. There can be little doubt that the type and extent of past experience both with facilities and with users will have a strong bearing on salient beliefs and, ultimately, the willingness to accept facilities in the neighbourhood (Smith and Hanham, 1981). Given that community-based care is a relatively recent phenomenon in many places, neighbourhood facilities represent an unknown in many people's minds. This may engender a latent fear because of uncertainty, but is also likely to mean that beliefs will change once first-hand experience has been gained. The nature of the experience will obviously determine whether such changes lead to more positive or more negative predispositions. Whether or not a particular individual or family member has received mental health care would seem an especially important influence on beliefs.

The third set of external variables included in the model consists of neighbourhood characteristics, and here we distinguish between the physical and social structure of the neighbourhood. In terms of the first, land-use mix and environmental quality are perhaps especially important. For example, different beliefs about facility impacts seem likely in areas of mixed land use and low quality compared with high quality, wholly residential neighbourhoods. In the former a facility is less likely to be intrusive given the existing mixture of land uses and is also less likely to arouse beliefs about negative environmental consequences. The effects of the general social milieu of a neighbourhood on beliefs about the mentally ill and mental health facilities can be inferred from the work of Trute and Segal (1976). Their studies focussed on the social integration of mental health facilities in residential communities, and identified factors associated with varying levels of integration. Facilities with the highest levels of integration were in neighbourhoods of low social cohesion. These were characterized by a low proportion of married couples, high rates of single parent families and never-married and divorced individuals, a high proportion of older persons and people with low incomes, and a low proportion of homeowners. Social integration was low in highly cohesive neighbour-hoods, characteristic of suburban areas with a predominance of nuclear families and homogeneity of race, class, and educational background. Such neighbourhoods tended to close ranks against the incursion of the mentally ill. These findings suggest that the social structure affects individual beliefs about what the neighbourhood should be like and, consequently, beliefs about the suitability of the neighbourhood as a host for a mental health facility.

For clarity we have described the effects on beliefs of these different sets of external variables separately. In reality they operate in combination, and to assess the effects of any one variable it is important to take into account its interactions with all the other variables.

2.3.2 Salient beliefs

The second major component of the model comprises three sets of salient beliefs. These are beliefs about the impacts of facilities, beliefs about the mentally ill, and beliefs about the neighbourhood. The first set correspond to perceptions of the external effects of facilities. As shown in the first section of this chapter, considerable importance is attached to externality effects in public facility location theory. With reference to the analysis of community response to facilities, it is the subjective assessment of the potential or actual externalities by local residents which is of prime concern. Beliefs about the effects that a facility might have or is having are what count, even if these beliefs do not accord very well with reality. Beliefs about the negative effects of facilities on property values are a good example of this. They frequently emerge as a strong motivation for opposing a facility location, and yet there is little if any empirical evidence to show that a property value decline actually occurs (see chapter 9). Previous research provides some basis for identifying the range of perceived external effects that might underlie salient beliefs about neighbourhood mental health facilities. We can distinguish between tangible and intangible effects. The former are related to specific characteristics of the facility and its operation such as the size and design of the building. The latter are more subjective and include concerns about personal safety, neighbourhood image, and environmental quality.

Community response to mental health facilities is almost certainly more a response to the users than to the facility itself. For this reason we regard beliefs about the mentally ill to be a vital component of the model. We can benefit greatly from the extensive previous research which has investigated public opinions about the mentally ill and particularly from the scaling instruments that this provides. At the same time we recognize that much of this research predates the community mental health movement and was undertaken largely in the context of hospital-based care. It seems extremely important, therefore, to revise existing instruments or to devise new ones to ensure the measures obtained are relevant to current modes of service delivery. To this end in our research (see chapter 6), we develop a new set of scales taking as a starting point the work of Cohen and Struening (1962) and Baker and Schulberg (1967). In previous research the term 'attitudes' has normally been used with reference to public sentiments about the mentally ill. The concepts actually measured by existing scales are, however, more accurately termed 'beliefs' given that the statements that make up these scales typically comprise various expressions of belief about the characteristics of the mentally ill and of the treatment they should receive. We prefer to limit the term 'attitudes' to evaluative judgements of positive or negative effects which, though based upon beliefs, are not synonymous with them.

We include beliefs about the neighbourhood as a third set of salient beliefs. Community response to a facility is likely to be significantly influenced by the type of neighbourhood in which it is located. Local residents hold beliefs about the characteristics that their neighbourhood should have, and it is in light of these that the suitability of a facility location is evaluated. Neighbourhood and facility beliefs therefore interact to determine the perceived 'fit' of a particular facility in a given neighbourhood. A wide range of neighbourhood beliefs potentially contribute to the assessment of fit. They encompass perceptions of the physical and social characteristics of the neighbourhood.

We do not explicitly incorporate within the model the distinction between behavioural and normative beliefs which Fishbein and Ajzen make in their theory of reasoned action. We do, however, acknowledge that the origin of salient beliefs is to a varying extent dependent upon social influences. Certain beliefs may be quite idiosyncratic and therefore largely personal; others may be shared by many within the same community and may have been acquired by any one individual through social contact. The contribution of social influences deserves emphasis. Although our model is constructed at the individual level, we recognize that individual attitudes and behaviour are strongly influenced by contextual factors and possibly nowhere more so than in the role played by normative beliefs.

2.3.3 Attitudes

The three sets of salient beliefs are the foundation for the formation of attitudes. In the previous section we pointed out the important distinction between attitudes toward objects, and attitudes toward behaviour with respect to those objects. Where our concern is with the prediction and explanation of single actions, our focus has to be on attitudes toward behaviour if we hope to show strong attitude–behaviour relationships. On the other hand, if we are concerned with overall patterns of behaviour we may legitimately consider attitudes toward the objects of that behaviour as relevant antecedents. In our case, concern focusses on explaining patterns of behaviour with respect to neighbourhood mental health facilities and their implications for community acceptance or rejection of facilities. For this reason we choose to focus on attitudes toward facilities as the attitudinal component of our model, rather than on attitudes toward undertaking specific behaviours. We acknowedge that if our objectives were more narrowly defined, a restricted concept of attitudes would be appropriate. Notice, however, that our use of attitudes is consistent with the treatment of beliefs just described. We described beliefs about objects (neighbourhood mental health facility, the mentally ill, and the neighbourhood) and not about behaviour. Within the model, therefore, attitudes represent an individual's overall subjective evaluation of community mental health facilities, and the extent to which he or she is positively or negatively disposed toward them.

2.3.4 Behavioural intentions
The focus on general patterns of behaviour rather than single actions also has a direct bearing on our treatment of behavioural intentions, the next component of the model. We are not concerned with the intention to undertake any one behaviour, but rather with intentions to participate in a range of behaviours considered in combination. The latter provide a more complete indication of potential behavioural patterns than reliance on a single behavioural intention. In broad terms, behavioural intentions fall into three groups: those supportive of a facility, those opposed, and those which are neutral. The last may simply be the intention to do nothing. Previous research on community response to public facilities has tended to concentrate on oppositional behaviour and the distinction has been made between intentions to undertake individual and group actions (Taylor and Hall, 1977). The former include writing to a newspaper, contacting a local official, and moving house; the latter comprise such actions as signing a petition, attending a meeting, and joining a protest group. A simple index of behavioural intentions can be calculated from the number of actions any individual intends. It may be appropriate to apply differential weights to reflect the seriousness of different behaviours. The model proposes a strong link between an individual's attitude toward a facility and a general index of behavioural intentions.

2.3.5 Behaviour
Behavioural intentions are the immediate antecedents of behaviour. The link between the two assumes that individuals behave in a rational manner, and that actions are not a function of unconscious or random forces, but are based on definite intentions. It would perhaps be difficult to support this view for all behaviours, but not for those which are our focus of concern. Actions taken with respect to community mental health facilities can be reasonably assumed to follow from careful consideration, and to reflect deliberate intentions.

The range of behaviours which are relevant to the analysis of community response to facilities correspond to those previously described with reference to intentions. A major problem, however, is to measure the occurrence of actual behaviour. Whereas in principle neighbourhood residents can indicate their behavioural intentions, they may have little

opportunity or reason to carry them out simply because their neighbourhood is not selected as a location for a facility. We would expect,
therefore, to have measures of actual behaviour for only a small proportion
of subjects in a study using a sample drawn from the general population.
The use of purposive samples drawn from areas where facility locations
are proposed, or already exist, can reduce this problem.

Measuring actual behaviour is also complicated because the time of
occurrence is often hard to anticipate. An individual may indicate an
intention to write to a newspaper about a neighbourhood facility, but the
time period within which this action could occur may remain undefined.
To begin with, the intention may be conditional upon a facility location
being proposed, but, even if this is certain, undertaking the behaviour may
still occur at any time over a relatively extensive period. A partial solution
to this problem lies in making the measures of behavioural intentions as
specific as possible. Ajzen and Fishbein (1980) stress the need to specify
the following for each intention: the intended action, the target of the
action, the context, and the time period. For the previous example, the
intended action is writing to the newspaper, the target is the facility, the
context is the resident's neighbourhood, but the time period is unspecified.
The addition of appropriate time periods would place definite limits on the
length of time over which information on behaviour was required.

Another important point to recognize is that, in general, the longer the
time lapse between the measurement of intentions and the occurrence
of behaviour, the weaker the relationship between the two is likely to be,
because intentions may have changed in the interim. These problems are
most serious when the objective is to predict single actions by an individual.
They are likely to be of less concern when the focus is on general patterns
of behaviour, especially if the units of analysis are aggregates rather than
individuals. As previously indicated, this is commonly the case in studies
of community response to facilities. Ajzen and Fishbein (1980) point to
the considerable evidence which shows that even when predictions of
behaviour from intentions are poor at the individual level, they are often
remarkably accurate at the aggregate level.

2.3.6 Outcomes
The final component of the model is the outcome of facility acceptance
or rejection. Notice that acceptance or rejection is not a behaviour but a
product of behaviour. In fact, one or more of several behaviours within
the sets of actions associated with support for, or opposition to, a facility
can lead to either outcome. Rarely will the outcome be the result of the
action of a single individual. Most often a combination of actions by groups
of individuals are involved. Moreover, the characteristics of the groups
(for example, political power and influence) involved will have an
important bearing on the effectiveness of actions to achieve desired
outcomes.

The outcome resulting from particular actions is not always obvious, and this is especially true for relatively neutral behaviours. For example, is taking no action (either to support or to oppose a facility) linked to acceptance or rejection? Does indifference represent silent opposition or marginal support? These are important questions, since it is likely that the majority in any community will be inactive. On the other hand, it may be sensible to concentrate on the behaviours of the active minority since these may be decisive in determining the final outcome. But there may still be complications if different minority groups within the same community act in different ways such that some sort of balance of power determines the outcome. The link between behaviour and outcome is therefore not as self-evident as it might at first appear.

The potential for ambiguity in defining outcomes has important implications for locational decisions. For example, faced with apparent widespread indifference within a community or with conflict between different groups, a local authority has to gauge what the final outcome of a facility location would be. This may be a very difficult judgement to make. One approach to this problem is for planners to try and shape the course of events through the use of information and education programs designed to promote a positive response to a proposed facility. This strategy potentially provides a forum within which ambiguities can be resolved and the likelihood of particular outcomes made more certain. This type of intervention is one example of how extraneous factors may affect eventual outcomes. The prediction and explanation of facility acceptance or rejection may therefore not depend solely on the behaviours of community residents. For this reason, the analysis of outcomes is more complicated than the study of behaviour.

2.3.7 The relationship between individual and aggregate response
At this point we need to clarify the relationship between individual and aggregate response to facilities. As described, the model identifies the factors affecting the behaviour of an individual in response to a facility location. At the same time, we have indicated that the eventual outcome of facility acceptance or rejection normally depends upon the actions of groups rather than single individuals. This implies that individuals typically join forces to translate their behavioural intentions into actions, and that subsequent outcomes are dependent upon the characteristics of the collective action. The formation of groups comprising individuals with beliefs, attitudes, and intentions is an intrinsic part of the political process involved in locating public facilities.

The reasons that like-minded individuals form groups as the basis for action are reasonably clear. Group action is both a more efficient and a potentially more effective way of communicating public concerns over local issues than sporadic, uncoordinated efforts by separate individuals.

Group actions are less easily ignored by those in authority. Collective opposition almost always poses a greater threat [see Olson (1965) for a full discussion]. The reasons for collective action are of less concern in the present context than are the characteristics of social groups which affect outcomes. In this regard, political power and influence is especially important.

It is well known that different social groups within society vary in their political power and influence. In large measure, these variations coincide with social class stratification. Each group is motivated primarily by the self-interests of its members. In the urban context, these interests commonly involve groups competing to attract desirable resources into, and keep undesirable resources out of, their neighbourhoods. Herein lie the roots of community-based conflict over the provision of urban services and amenities [see Harvey (1973) and Castells (1978) for detailed discussion of these issues]. Neighbourhood mental health facilities are usually regarded as unwanted, if necessary, services. In general, therefore, we can expect neighbourhood groups to resist their location. Resistance inevitably involves participation in the political process. This can take various forms including the formation of action groups, attendance at public meetings, lobbying elected officials, etc. The extent to which this participation succeeds in achieving the group's objectives depends to a large degree on the access which the group has to those in authority. Middle and upper class groups tend to have better access and influence because they are often better organized and more able to communicate their concerns effectively, and because those in authority are commonly from these groups and are concerned to protect their own self-interests by acceding to the group's desires. This is an oversimplification of a complex political process, but it suffices for present purposes because it reveals that group-based action has important implications for the link between behaviour and outcomes within the model.

The major implication is that the outcomes resulting from behaviour will depend on the political power and influence of the group through which the behaviour is channelled. It is conceivable that the same behaviour performed by separate individuals within different social groups will achieve very different results. This underlies the point made earlier that, with respect to the prediction and explanation of outcomes, it is very important to identify and take account of salient extraneous factors in addition to the measures of relevant behaviour.

The political power vested in different social groups is especially important for understanding the outcomes of community response to mental health facilities. In our empirical analysis this is not a major focus because we concentrate more on the relationships leading to individual behavioural intentions. Nonetheless, the importance of group-based factors has to be kept in mind and we recognize this by the inclusion of neighbourhood contextual variables within the set of external variables

affecting belief formation. We must note also that the outcomes of
group-based action have direct implications for the future intentions of
individual group members. Success in achieving the group's objectives is
likely to strengthen the intentions of its members to behave in the same
way should a similar situation arise at a future point. Failure, on the
other hand, may cause a reassessment of intentions, and thereby change
behaviour on a subsequent occasion. Relating these feedback effects to
status-based variations in group power implies that the more successful
middle and upper status groups will continue to be effective, whereas the
less successful lower status groups may well weaken in their resolve and
slip into apathetic and resigned acceptance of unwanted conditions. We
see, therefore, that individual response to mental health facilities cannot
be examined in isolation from aggregate behaviour. We need to recognize
that the two interact and that an understanding of these interactions is
basic to an explanation of facility acceptance or rejection.

2.4 Conclusions

In this chapter we have drawn upon public facility location theory and the
theory of attitude formation to develop a theoretical model for our
investigation of community response to mental health facilities. Public
facility location theory identifies the importance of the spatial externalities
of locational decisions. In the case of mental health facility locations,
these externalities are often perceived negatively by nonusers in the
surrounding community and contribute to the development of negative
public attitudes and behavioural reactions. The process which underlies
attitude formation and behavioural responses can be analyzed within the
framework of the theory of reasoned action proposed by Fishbein and
Ajzen. The theory postulates a sequential process in which attitudes play
a central role linking various sets of external variables and salient beliefs
with behavioural intentions and behaviour.

The model which we developed based on the Fishbein–Ajzen framework
contains three sets of external variables: facility–user characteristics,
personal characteristics, and neighbourhood characteristics. These are
linked to three sets of salient beliefs regarding facility impacts, the mentally
ill, and the neighbourhood, which together are the antecedents of attitudes
toward facilities. Behavioural intentions are based on these attitudes and
intentions are linked directly to behaviour. The model is developed to
describe the formation of attitudes and behavioural intentions at the
individual level. We recognize, however, that behaviour is typically an
aggregate phenomenon involving group-based action. Equally, the outcomes
of behaviour, in terms of facility acceptance or rejection, depend to a
great extent on the characteristics of the groups involved, particularly
their political power and influence. The ways in which the attitudes and
intentions of different individuals interact and fuse to form the basis for

collective action are complex, but have to be understood if community response to facilities is to be explained.

One further point needs to be made. We are acutely aware of the epistemological problems of linking models of individual behaviour (from attitude theory) with models of aggregate social process (from public facility location theory). We have not achieved a complete articulation between these two modes of analysis in this research. On the one hand, the behavioural model (figure 2.1) provides a comprehensive theorization of individual response, including a range of external variables representing the social context. On the other hand, we have not provided a full explanation of how belief systems are engendered and structured within that context. Our research bias toward the former analytical model is defensible in the light of our stated research goal of establishing community attitudes toward the mentally ill and mental health facilities. The task of fully articulating our findings with a more structuralist view of social process must be undertaken at a later date. It would require a comprehensive theory of the production and reproduction of urban social space, especially neighbourhoods, of the kind developed in Scott (1980); and it would need to clarify how the mentally ill intervene in the reproduction process so as to cause their rejection by threatened neighbourhoods—a complex process tentatively described in Dear (1981). Until such time as this synthesis can be made, we are content to outline the broad interrelationship between our model and the wider social context. This occurs in the examination of society and state in the historical development of mental health policy (chapter 3); in the question of community stake and status in the development of neighbourhood attitudes (chapter 8); and in the broad schema for neighbourhood acceptance and rejection of mental health facilities (chapter 10).

A social history of the asylum

The purpose of this chapter is to provide a brief overview of the social history of the asylum. This is the first of two chapters which provide the background to our investigation of community attitudes toward the mentally ill and mental health facilities. Contemporary attitudes need to be set in the context of society's treatment of the mentally ill in the past. We focus on the 'social' history of the asylum, since it is not part of our concern to examine the technical aspects of treatment nor of the administrative growth of the psychiatric profession. Instead, we wish to explore the growth of mental health care in its social context, in order to understand the link between society and mental illness and the genesis of contemporary social attitudes toward the mentally ill (see chapter 4).

Mental illness and mental health care are fields of intense and continuing controversy. In historical terms, many critics have attempted to map the "geography of [these] haunted places" (Foucault, 1973, page 57), beginning with the loosening of the lunatic's chains and ending with the birth of the asylum. Contemporary scholars have turned their attention to the increasing penetration of the psychiatric profession into everyday living. This attempt to 'psychiatrize' a wide range of social problems is viewed with growing scepticism, and many view with suspicion the seemingly crude methods of psychiatric treatment, including electroconvulsive therapy and involuntary commitment (Clare, 1976).

The history of mental health care is a study in isolation and exclusion. Every culture appears to have had its 'madness', and to have found some method of isolating the mentally ill. These methods have sometimes been crude (as when the mad were forced to live beyond the confines of mediaeval towns), and often well-intentioned (as with the development of the asylum—a true place of refuge). In all situations, however, the response has been to isolate and to exclude. The history which we review in this chapter explores the diverse means of exclusion. It is not a complex history, although there is much diversity in detail; instead, we shall witness a constant cycle of psychiatric philosophies, as the caring professions swing regularly between the poles of 'conscience' and 'convenience', in Rothman's phrasing (Rothman, 1980; see also Allderidge, 1979).

3.1 The general argument

Most societies seem to have recognized certain extreme forms of aberrant behaviour as evidence of mental instability or insanity. The point at which, along a continuum of human behaviour, an individual is regarded as mad will depend upon various factors. These include the characteristics of the aberrant behaviour, its style and consistency, and its consequences. However, a second set of factors involves the extent to which a society will tolerate eccentric behaviour, and is reflected in the kinds of social institution designed to 'treat' the deviant individual. Whether or not a person is considered mad, therefore, depends upon the degree of behavioural disturbance *and* the attitudes of society toward deviant behaviour. Hence, 'mental disorder' in any society is intimately linked to social factors as well as to illness-related considerations. The key to understanding mental illness lies not only in the impaired individuals, but also in understanding the perceptual and social environment in which they exist.

After an extensive review of definitions of mental health, Clare (1976) can only conclude that most definitions embody a strong social value in their content. He summarizes his frustration ironically as follows:

"The mentally healthy person is not a nuisance, does not challenge the rules, lose his temper, kick the cat, or park his car [illegally]. He makes no demands, passes his life quietly and productively and does not fiddle the social security, live with a mistress, or wear placards warning that the end of the world is nigh" (Clare, 1976, page 15).

This ever-changing, 'negotiated' character of mental illness is a central theme in this chapter. We shall show how the social history of the asylum is a mirror of the contemporary socioeconomic milieu (D'Arcy, 1976). Since, of necessity, any social history must be culture-specific, the saga which unfolds here is limited to developments within Western Europe and North America. Within these two continents, the patterns of care have not been homogeneous; however, the general themes which we wish to pursue are universally applicable. A more detailed survey of the Ontario experience concludes this chapter, to set the scene for the later analysis.

3.2 Early history: the period of classical antiquity in Greece and Rome

From his survey of the status of the mentally ill in Greece and Rome, Rosen (1968, chapter 3) concludes that the problem of madness was handled largely on the basis of custom. Greek medicine had earlier rejected any supernatural explanation of mental disorder, although popular belief both in Greece and in Rome held that mental abnormality was due to some supernatural power which entered the body or produced its effect by action from without. This idea had ancient roots, for Plato had proposed that atheists, whose lack of faith derived from ignorance and not malice, should be placed in a 'house of sanity' for five years (Simon, 1978, page 32).

By the fifth century BC, a variety of attitudes toward the mentally ill had developed, although religious fear and awe still strongly influenced common perceptions. These attitudes mingled fear of violent behaviour with contempt for individuals lacking the normal sensibilities of human beings. An element of comparison was also present, for although the mentally disabled became objects of scorn and amusement, no effort was made to conceal the mad. They were a visible part of everyday experience.

Hence, in Graeco–Roman antiquity, it was possible for mentally disabled individuals to function in society as long as their behavioural impairment brought no harm to themselves or to society. Moreover, as Rosen (1968, page 109) observes, certain "... culturally constituted systems, particularly religious beliefs and practices, provided a means by which individuals might effectively achieve some form of adjustment to society".

For the most part, actual *care* of the mentally ill was left to their friends and relatives. No asylums or special institutions for the treatment or custody of the mentally ill existed. There were, of course, institutional arrangements for custodial care of the violent mad. However, Graeco–Roman society seems to have cared less about the nature and cause of insanity, and more about demonstrating unsoundness of mind and its consequences in behaviour. Given the variety of attitudes toward mental illness, it is not surprising that many treatment methods for the mentally ill were attempted. For those who could afford it, medical treatment by a doctor was possible. This could include physical cures, such as bleeding; alternatively, early efforts at the psychotherapeutic approach were possible when enlightened physicians recognized the importance of psychological factors (for example, grief) in causing mental illness. Generally, however, neither physician nor community played a major role in care of the mentally ill in Greece and Rome. Many insane resorted to religious or magical treatment because of the confusion over the etiology of mental illness, or because previous 'cures' had failed.

3.3 The roots of the asylum
Concepts of mental illness in Mediaeval Europe derived largely from the ideas of classical antiquity, and were only slowly modified by subsequent events (Rosen, 1968, chapter 4). During this period, public authorities took only limited responsibility for the mentally disabled, who remained at liberty as long as they caused no public disturbance. A large amount of disturbance in this period was due to theological dogma and popular beliefs regarding demonic possession and witchcraft, creating a new class of social deviants who were mercilessly pursued.

As before, responsibility for the custody of the mentally ill rested with relatives and friends. However, those who were too dangerous, or lacked someone to care for them, were cared for by communal authorities. Despite much local variation, the principle of limited public responsibility for the mentally ill was widely accepted throughout western and central Europe by the middle of the fifteenth century. Acutely disturbed patients were often admitted to general hospitals, as, for example, at the Hôtel-Dieu in Paris, and in other parts of Germany and England. In light of the general principle of caring for one's own, many insane who were native to other communities were frequently expelled and returned to their original community.

By the end of the sixteenth century in Europe, there was a discernible trend toward placing the mentally disabled into some form of institution-based care. For instance, former leper houses were converted to house the insane (Rosen, 1968, page 142). An important precedent for this tendency toward confinement was the practice of excluding the insane from towns, which was especially frequent in fifteenth-century Germany (Foucault, 1973, chapter 1). They were allowed to wander in the open countryside when not entrusted to a group of merchants or pilgrims. Frequently, the mad were handed over to boatmen, who then disembarked with their 'ship of fools', ultimately intending to drop off their cargo in uninhabited places.

Scarcely a century after the mad ships we encounter the madhouse, or asylum. The purely negative measures of exclusion are totally replaced by principles of confinement. In these tendencies toward exclusion and confinement, against the background of social upheaval in Renaissance Europe, the roots of the asylum may be perceived.

3.4 The birth of the asylum
The birth of the asylum in Europe and North America in the seventeenth and eighteenth centuries is essentially a history of the principle of confinement.

3.4.1 Europe
In seventeenth-century and eighteenth-century Europe, mental illness was progressively removed from the social scene. Following significant shifts in social attitudes, the mentally disabled became a community responsibility. The most important contributory factor in changing attitudes was the increasing burden of the poor and indigent upon local community resources (Rosen, 1968, chapter 5). To deal with the problems of the poor, the dependent, and the deviant, enormous 'houses of confinement' were created in the seventeenth century (Foucault, 1973, chapter 2). A policy of internment and indoor relief was adopted and institutions were created to put the policy into practice. The outstanding landmark of this trend was the founding of the Hôpital Général in Paris, in 1656. This was not a medical establishment. Its purposes were economic, social, moral. It was intended to increase manufactures, provide productive work, and end unemployment; to punish idleness, restore public order, and rid Paris of beggars; and to relieve the needy, deal with immorality and antisocial behaviour, and provide Christian instruction (Rosen, 1968, pages 162–163). Within several months of its opening, more than one out of every one hundred inhabitants of Paris found themselves confined within the Hôpital Général (a total of 6000 people). These included the old, those with venereal disease, epileptics, and the mentally ill. In segregating deviants by internment, the hospital combined the characteristics of a penal institution, an asylum, a workhouse, and a medical facility.

According to Foucault, the house of confinement in Europe replaced the leprosaria (which had developed about 1100–1300 AD) in the 'geography of haunted places'. He emphasizes the link between mental health policy and the contemporary economic crises of western Europe:

"For a long time, the house of correction or the premises of the Hôpital Général would serve to contain the unemployed, the idle, and vagabonds. Each time a crisis occurred and the number of poor sharply increased, the houses of confinement regained ... their initial economic significance.

But outside of the periods of crisis, confinement acquired another meaning. Its repressive function was combined with a new use. It was no longer merely a question of confining those out of work, but of giving work to those who had been confined and thus making them contribute to the prosperity of all. The alternation is clear: cheap manpower in the periods of full employment and high salaries; and in periods of unemployment, reabsorption of the idle and social protection against agitation and uprising" (Foucault, 1973, pages 50–51).

By the end of the seventeenth century, therefore, we are observing much more than a simple evolution of social institutions. Madness was now irrevocably linked to the consequences of historical development and a changing social environment. All forms of social uselessness were rejected by society, and the institutions to facilitate this ideology had been created (Donzelot, 1979).

During the eighteenth century, the conditions in the institutions of confinement deteriorated rapidly. They were usually grossly overcrowded, and the mélange of inmates created new problems. Only one-tenth of those confined in the Paris Hôpital Général were described as 'insane', and mad and sane mingled together freely. The possibility of 'treatment' was not considered (Foucault, 1973, chapter 3; Rosen, 1968, chapter 5). Conditions were so bad that, during the second half of the eighteenth century, a new reform movement was begun. Its objective was not to suppress the institutions of confinement, but to neutralize them as potential causes of new social ills. Henceforth, confinement was to be reserved for criminals and the insane, and special institutions were to be created to segregate and care for the mentally ill. This social movement represented the true birth of the insane asylum (Foucault, 1973, chapters 7 and 8).

The philosophical basis of a separate asylum for the insane has its origins in what we would now call the principles of 'social psychiatry'. Broadly speaking, these principles assert the link between social environment and mental illness. For example, the effect of wars and revolution in increasing psychoses had already been noted by the time of the French revolution. Hence, if mental illness was induced by conditions of society, then mental health could be encouraged by removal of the sufferer from the source of irritation. A major experiment in the care and treatment of the mentally ill was the founding of the Retreat, in York, England, by the Society of

Friends in 1796. This project was conceived by William Tuke, and was based on a regimen of humane treatment (good food, exercise, occupation) and Christianity. Almost simultaneously, Phillippe Pinel was introducing a system of 'moral treatment' at the Bicêtre and Salpêtrière asylums in Paris. Here the removal of mechanical restraints proved the value of humane treatment of the mentally ill. These invaluable experiences had a profound effect throughout Europe and North America. The model for special institutions for the mentally disabled had been established.

3.4.2 America

There is no evidence that mental illness was widespread in colonial America, and virtually none of the legislation enacted by colonial legislatures addressed the treatment of the insane (Grob, 1973, chapter 1). Not until the late seventeenth and eighteenth century did demographic changes force an alteration in the pattern of welfare and encourage the institutionalization of the mentally disabled. By 1773, the State of Virginia had established the first hospital devoted exclusively to the care and treatment of the mentally ill in America, although (as in Europe) the insane had previously been confined in other institutions.

To understand the discovery and proliferation of the asylum in eighteenth-century America, it is essential to recognize that, at this period,

"Psychiatrists were more American than they were scientific, and the nature of their response to insanity cannot be comprehended unless one recognizes that they defined mental illness as a social problem, not just a medical one ... prisons, poorhouses, and orphan asylums grew up at the same time, and this coincidence suggests that the society was reacting to more than psychiatric doctrines" (Rothman, 1971, page xv).

The birth of the asylum in the Jacksonian period was nothing less than a vigorous attempt, on many fronts, to promote the stability of society at a time of flux. Perhaps more than their European counterparts, American physicians closely linked the etiology of mental illness to social conditions, focussing especially upon the effect of a 'startlingly fluid' social order, religious excess, and conditions of schooling, family, and heredity (Rothman, 1971, chapter 5). This emphasis on family and community reinforced the concept of treatment involving a specially created, and therefore corruption-free, setting for the deviant:

"The distinctive environment which would eliminate the threat to the American social order was the asylum, which therefore acquired an enormously significant fusion of morality and law. The asylum was to fulfill a dual purpose for its innovators. It would rehabilitate inmates and then, by virtue of its success, set an example of right action for the larger society .... Just as the penitentiary would reform the criminal and the insane asylum would cure the mentally ill, so the almshouse would rehabilitate the poor" (Rothman, 1971, pages xix and 180).

3.5 Nineteenth-century consolidation and growth

At the beginning of the nineteenth century, the stage was set for the expansion and consolidation of the asylum philosophy in Europe and America. (The same was true of Canada which, being a younger country, lagged behind its continental neighbour.) The history of the transition from nineteenth-century optimism to the twentieth-century revolution in mental health care related in this section concentrates mainly upon America, although parallel stories may be told for Canada and Europe (Jones, 1972).

The care and treatment of the insane in nineteenth-century America was based on a philosophy which fused morality, social values, and science (Grob, 1973, chapter 4). Most psychiatrists were convinced that insanity could be cured, and that confinement in an institution so that medical and (more especially) moral treatment could be administered was the keystone of the cure. The basic postulate of the asylum program was the prompt removal of the insane from the community to an institution which was itself separated from the community. A 'well-ordered institution' was believed to encourage social order in disorderly groups (Rothman, 1971, chapter 6).

During the first quarter of the nineteenth century, much of the hospital movement was a product of private philanthropy. However, by the middle of the century, an extensive network of state-supported public hospitals had been established. In 1860, most states had at least one hospital for the care of the mentally ill (Grob, 1973, chapter 3). The hospitals were administered by a centralized state authority, which soon became the vehicle by which the state imposed a centralized, rationalized, bureaucratic framework upon its welfare institutions. This bureaucracy was to aggravate the problems of growth which beset the asylum system in the latter half of the nineteenth century.

In the years that succeeded the establishment of a comprehensive system of public asylums, the gap between the ideal model of a mental hospital and the social reality steadily widened. As the problems of asylum management multiplied, the objective of rehabilitation through moral treatment declined to one of simple custodianship. A large variety of reasons have been offered to account for this change (Grob, 1973, chapter 5; Rothman, 1971, chapter 10). These include a set of internal and external considerations. The former crystallize around the massive pressure on the asylum to accommodate more and more patients as the size of the general population expanded. Careful treatment of these inflated patient populations became virtually impossible, and early optimism about 'cure' was lost. This factor was aggravated as hospitals became saturated by chronic patients who were not responsive to treatment. The latter group of external considerations exacerbated the dilemmas of growth in the asylums; especially significant were the escalating costs of asylums in the latter half of the nineteenth century. Between 1870 and 1880, nearly thirty new institutions were opened in America. However, incarceration was now principally a means of controlling deviant and dependent populations. As Rothman (1971, page 240) points out: "The promise of reform had built up the asylums; the functionalism of custody perpetuated them".

One of the by-products of the founding of mental hospitals in America in the eighteenth and nineteenth centuries was the birth of the psychiatric profession (Grob, 1973, chapter 4). Irrespective of claims of its scientific or medical character, psychiatry reflected the role assigned to it by society and, hence, mirrored the dominant values of that society. Thus, by the 1840s, a self-conscious profession, confident of its unique expertise, had emerged within the more general framework of welfare and dependency. The hospitals were managed by superintendents—psychiatrists who were frequently lay people or were selected from a corpus of socially concerned physicians. In 1844, a group of thirteen of the most distinguished superintendents met in Philadelphia and founded the Association of Medical Superintendents of American Institutions for the Insane (AMSAII, now the American Psychiatric Association). The AMSAII prepared guidelines to govern the care and treatment of the mentally ill. They argued, amongst other things, that mental illness "... was fundamentally no different from physical illness; it therefore required trained and experienced personnel" (Grob, 1973, page 138). They laid emphasis on a broad range of physical, mental, and moral factors in the etiology of mental illness (Deutsch, 1949). This eclecticism is, of course, quite understandable, given the climate of uncertainty in psychiatric diagnosis and the absence of specifically demonstrable causal etiological links. Moreover, the homogenous social background and mixed training of the superintendents tended to detract from a purely medical interpretation of mental illness (Grob, 1973, pages 153–159).

The most complex organizational problem facing the fledgling AMSAII was its wider relationship with the medical profession generally. Although the superintendents viewed insanity as a 'disease', they were highly reluctant to affiliate with the American Medical Association (AMA) which was founded three years later in 1847. An AMSAII motion proposing affiliation was soundly defeated in 1853, and all subsequent efforts at amalgamation proved futile. Although a major factor in this rejection was psychiatrists' fear that their independence and power would be threatened by affiliation with the AMA, many were also sensitive to the precipitous decline in the status of the American medical profession in the nineteenth century (Grob, 1973, page 149). The absence of state licensing legislation had caused a proliferation of medical 'sects' at the same time as 'doctors' were daily demonstrating a manifest inability to deal with disease. The consequent withering of public confidence did nothing to inspire the AMSAII of the virtue of professional affiliation! This antipathy was compounded by the increasingly 'administrative' character which the psychiatric profession took upon itself in the 1860s and thereafter.

Admission to the profession depended less upon specialized training and more upon actual experience in mental hospitals.

Later in the nineteenth century, the antagonism between the AMSAII and the AMA again flared up. The focus of controversy was the debate over the need for separate facilities for the treatment of the 'incurable' mentally ill. As mental hospitals became increasingly overcrowded, and the revitalized medical profession took a fresh interest in the insane, Dr S D Willard (secretary of the Medical Society of the State of New York) prepared a report for the New York legislature on the conditions of the insane poor in the state. The report concluded by recommending the establishment of a new institution for incurables in order to relieve local welfare institutions. The legislature concurred with this proposal and, in 1869, the Willard Asylum for the Insane opened for the reception of chronic cases. This action was a direct affront to many mental hospital superintendents, since the legislation was counter to their professional judgement (Grob, 1973, pages 309–319). This conflict of interest caused a split within the AMSAII and generated much inconclusive interprofessional dispute. It remained one of the most important factors in the AMSAIIs continuing refusal to merge with the AMA (Rothman, 1971, page 282).

It is instructive to compare briefly the experience of American psychiatry with the rise of the psychiatric profession in Britain. Scull (1978) has documented the increasing attempts which were made from the mid-eighteenth century to claim insanity as part of the legitimate domain of medicine. In Britain, this claim was initially based in the most precarious of philosophies since the success of 'moral treatment' in Britain diminished the importance of traditional medicine. Moral treatment had been developed by lay people, and the model of William Tuke's lay-run Retreat at York dominated the public imagination (Jones, 1972). The problem of how to accommodate mental treatment within the general rubric of medicine caused a spate of books and pamphlets to appear in the early eighteenth century, often blaming the stories of disrepute in asylums on the absence of physician control in those institutions. In a spirit of compromise, a combination of moral and physical treatment was ultimately advocated and increasingly accepted. This had the effect of leaving the physician in control of the asylum by dint of his specialist knowledge. By the 1830s almost all public mental hospitals had a resident medical director. One of the first moves to consolidate the internal status arrangements of the new profession was the founding, in 1841, of the Association of Medical Officers of Asylums and Hospitals for the Insane. The Association, and its affiliated professional publications, emphasized insanity as a disease of the brain.

From its earliest inception, therefore, British psychiatry had tended to be dominated by the medical profession, and has been encouraged to think in terms of the medical model. These trends, which differ

significantly from those in America, were undoubtedly fostered by the
strength of the medical profession in Britain. The first College of
Physicians of London (later to become the Royal College of Physicians)
was founded in 1518. It was not until 1971 that a separate Royal College
of Psychiatrists was established, giving the profession independence in
setting standards for entry to the profession, examinations, and official
advisory capacity to the national government. Before 1971, these functions
were the responsibility of the Royal College of Physicians (Rosenzweig,
1975, chapter 4).

3.6 Deinstitutionalization and the community mental health movement

By the end of the nineteenth century, as asylums became increasingly
custodial and desparately overcrowded, new philosophies were sought.
Rothman (1980) describes this progressive era in America as a constant
struggle between 'conscience' and 'convenience', with the latter usually
winning. Indeed, until the middle of the twentieth century, the institution
of the asylum dominated the pattern of psychiatric care. This was in
spite of a burgeoning 'mental hygiene' movement which sought to promote
mental health in a noninstitutional setting. Mental health, it was argued,
could be achieved through hospitals which would seek cures to mental
illness, arrangements for postinstitutional care, and educational programs.
However, as the mental health industry became more complex, it was the
asylum which endured. The efforts at prevention and community out-
reach foundered on the institutional monolith (Rothman, 1980, chapters 9
and 10; also Magaro et al, 1978, chapter 2).

The patterns of nineteenth-century care continued essentially undisturbed;
any innovations usually became supplements to the system, and not
replacements. However, the seeds of community-based mental health had
taken hold in the mental hygiene movement [Allderidge (1979) would
argue that they already existed in previous centuries]. Since 1945, the
pace of change in mental health care has accelerated rapidly, so that it is
possible to speak of the 'revolution' in mental health care which occurred
during the third quarter of the twentieth century. This is usually referred
to as the 'community mental health' movement.

After World War 2, significant changes in public attitudes toward mental
illness were evident. The need to treat disorders of the returning war
veterans was coupled with a new awareness of the extent of mental
disabilities. For instance, of the five million men rejected from the US
draft because of failure to meet medical standards, some 40% were excluded
because of neuropsychiatric defects; moreover, such disabilities provided
the most frequent cause of discharge of those who were inducted but later
discharged for medical reasons (Beigel and Levinson, 1972, page 5). In
addition, national governments recognized the need to upgrade health and
welfare services which were neglected during the depression and war.

Hence, in Canada, the federal government instituted a series of National Health Grants in 1948 for the purpose of extending and improving public health and hospital services (Williams and Luterbach, 1976). In the United States a National Mental Health Act was passed in 1946, leading to the establishment of the National Institute of Mental Health in 1948 to administer a program of research, training, and service activities (Freedman, 1967). In Britain, major postwar reconstruction was being undertaken at the same time as experiments with the 'open hospital' system were underway.

It was in the 1950s that two developments occurred to revolutionize the treatment of the mentally ill. The first development, in Britain and later in North America, was the adoption of new psychosocial methods of treatment in the mental hospital. The methods focussed on the principles of 'social psychiatry', with its emphasis on avoidance of seclusion or of restraint, development of group techniques such as the therapeutic community, and so on. The second was the introduction of new tranquilizer drugs which contributed significantly to the effective treatment and symptomatic management of many psychotic patients. They also enabled reduction in the duration of hospital stays and increased the probability of discharge from hospital after chronic or acute episodes. As Klerman (1977) has indicated, the simultaneity of these two developments has obscured the relative contribution of drugs and hospital reform to the reduction of numbers of patients resident in asylums, and to the improved treatment outlook for the mentally ill. However, both developments, combined with changing public attitudes, prepared the way for deinstitutionalization and the community mental health movement of the 1960s.

Government response to the ferment for change was predictable. Commissions of inquiry were established in many countries to draft plans for the future of health services. The American experience in this respect is particularly instructive, since it has proceeded furthest. In 1955, the US Joint Congressional Commission on Mental Illness and Health began an exhaustive study of the mental health care delivery system. Their report criticized the concept of large state mental hospitals and advocated instead the development of services on a local basis. Under the impetus of the Kennedy administration, this philosophy was translated into the 1963 Community Mental Health Centers Act. The primary goal of this Act was to stimulate local communities to assume responsibility for the development of programs for care of their own mentally ill. Hence, federal funds were allocated to the construction and (later) the staffing of a nationwide system of comprehensive 'community mental health centers' (CMHC). Emphasis was placed upon the concept of community-based care since it was reasoned that the large state hospitals had done much to isolate the patient from society, to retard living skills, and to induce a level of disability and dependence over and above that arising from the patient's condition (Mechanic, 1969).

The impact of the CMHC program in the US has been enormous. The number of patients resident in state and county mental hospitals dropped from its 1955 peak of 559000 to 193000 in 1975. Prior to 1955, the hospital census was increasing at a rate of 2% per annum. As a result of this massive deinstitutionalization, many state hospitals have either closed or reduced their scale of operation. The percentage share of patient care episodes in mental hospitals (as a proportion of all care episodes) dropped from 49% in 1955 to 12% in 1973 (Bassuk and Gerson, 1978; National Institute of Mental Health, 1976). A major proportion of the reduction in the number of patients resident in public mental hospitals is accounted for by the movement of elderly patients from mental hospitals into nursing homes (Klerman, 1977, page 623). In addition, a major increase in the volume of services has occurred. The total number of inpatient and outpatient care episodes in all mental health facilities in 1945 was $1 \cdot 7$ million; by 1973 this had reached $5 \cdot 2$ million episodes. No less than 23% of these episodes occurred in community mental health centers. Although these national trends are evident in most states, there is (as is to be expected) considerable interstate variation in specific rates and trends (compare, Aviram et al, 1976).

The development of community-based mental health care has long been in evidence in Britain, though its evolution has been pragmatic and haphazard. The early legislation in this direction (the Mental Health Act of 1959) did little more than formalize a trend that had been developing for years. A notably successful experiment in community care had occurred in Worthing in the 1950s. Here, the medical superintendent of one hospital visited the homes of patients who had been referred for psychiatric hospitalization, and (by treatment and advice) enabled the patient to be cared for at home. In the final year of the 'Worthing Experiment', admissions to the hospital were reduced by 59%, even before the advent of psychotropic drugs. However, in Britain, as in America, the major reduction in mental hospital population occurred after the introduction of tranquilizers (Rosenzweig, 1975, chapter 3).

With the reduction in hospital populations, and concomitant increase in admission and (more especially) discharge rates, the care of the mentally ill in Britain moved de facto into the community. The resident population of mental hospitals in England and Wales dropped by 28% (to 103300) between 1951 and 1970 (Scull, 1978, page 70). It was not until 1962 that a Hospital Plan for England and Wales was published, confirming this trend, and announcing a sharp increase in the construction rate of community-based hospitals and other services (which were to be provided by the *local* government authorities). Although this shift toward local responsibility had been evident in the 1959 Act, local authorities have 'remained laggard' in assuming responsibility for community-based treatment of the mentally ill (Rosenzweig, 1975). Later government statements confirmed that the development of nonhospital, community-based facilities was an essential corollary of this plan. However, in reviewing these promised intentions in 1976, the *British Medical Journal* laments the "... virtual total absence of long-stay sheltered accommodation in the community" (17 January 1976, page 111). This 'limited progress' has been largely attributed to government failure to allocate the necessary funds toward the development of community resources. Clare (1976, pages 411–412)concludes:

"The running-down of the large mental hospitals has not been accompanied by a significant development of community based resources. Instead, there has been overcrowding in hospitals, a rise in the number of homeless and poorly housed people, and a shift of people from the mental health and into the prison services".

3.7 Mental health care in Ontario

The first care of the insane in North America was undertaken by the religious orders of New France (now the Province of Québec). Under direct intervention from France, the Hôtel Dieu of Québec was opened in 1639 "... for the care of indigent patients, the crippled and idiots" (Hurd, 1973, volume 1, page 446). It was not until 1835 that the first provincial institution for the care of the insane was established in St Johns, New Brunswick. Ontario, then known as Upper Canada, was the next to follow. In 1833, an act authorizing provincewide relief for 'destitute lunatics' was passed, and although it did not contemplate erecting an asylum, much effort in this direction was subsequently expended. Finally, in 1839, a grant of £3000 was authorized toward the erection of an asylum, and in 1841 the former York (Toronto) jail was outfitted as a temporary asylum (Hurd, 1973, volume 4, pages 120–130). A striking feature of the early history of asylums in Ontario is the extent to which 'branch' asylums developed, usually in response to overcrowding in existing institutions. Between 1840 and 1916, another ten public hospitals were erected, accommodating about 7000 people.

In 1867, the British North America Act assigned the responsibility for health, education, and social services to the Provinces. As in America, the early growth of services was dominated by asylums, which were essentially custodial in operation. The pattern of asylum growth largely reflected the general expansion of population, and the increasing number of beds served to maintain the bed : population ratio (Delottinville, 1976, chapter 2; Williams and Luterbach, 1976). Representative statistics of asylum growth in Ontario are shown in table 3.1. In spite of continuous expansion in bed capacity throughout the first half of this century, Ontario asylums were almost persistently overcrowded (Hanly, 1970; Richman, 1964, chapter 12).

Following 1945, the new awareness of mental illness prompted the federal government to institute a series of National Health Grants. The Mental Health Grant called on Provinces to assess their mental health needs.

The common theme of these individual provincial assessments was the
desire to "expand the existing structure and pattern of services" (Williams
and Luterbach, 1976, page 10). At least 80% of the 20051 psychiatric
beds authorized for construction between 1948 and 1961 were consigned,
as a consequence, to existing mental hospitals (Richman, 1964, chapter 3).
The custodial function thus endured.

In the face of continuing criticism, the federal government tried to
influence the direction of growth in psychiatric services, largely through
cost-sharing programs. However, significant changes in provincial practice
only came about after a flood of federal and provincial commissions on the
status of health services in Canada, for example, the Community Mental
Health Center Project (1972), and the Ontario Health Planning Task Force
(1974). These assessments, coupled with a bold attempt in Saskatchewan to
decentralize mental hospital services to smaller facilities (D'Arcy, 1976),
resulted in a strong move toward community-based mental health care.
The American model of a specific 'community mental health center' did
not materialize. Instead, Ontario, for instance, has worked toward
integrating psychiatric services with public health services. The thrust of
this effort has been directed toward integrating health, mental health, and
social services. Hence, community mental health care is often provided
from psychiatric units attached to general hospitals as well as from a
variety of outpatient units. Additional factors providing an impetus to
deinstitutionalization in Canada were the splitting off of special groups into
alternate forms of care (for example, geriatric patients and the mentally
retarded), a new stress on voluntary admissions, and the impact of new
drugs (Williams and Luterbach, 1976).

Table 3.1. Admissions, discharges, and 'on books' population of Ontario provincial
asylums for selected years, 1880–1976. (Sources: Annual Reports, Inspector of
Prisons and Public Charities, 1880–1940; Annual Report, Ontario Mental Hospitals,
1950–1976; Census of Canada, selected years.)

Year	Provincial population	Admissions	Discharges	'On books'[a]
1880	1923228	574	204	2899
1890	2114321	697	262	3955
1900	2182947	793	335	5877
1910	2572292	1140	555	6670
1920	2933662	2879	858	7689
1930	3431683	2469	1265	10390
1940	3787655	3224	2257	15283
1950	4597542	4334	2686	18923
1960	6236092	7820	6184	19507
1971	7703106	15712	15868	8838
1976	8264465	14112	14163	5030

[a] Before 1909, the 'on books' total is taken as the annual number of patients under
treatment.

The impact of these program developments on the pattern of care has been immense. In less than fifteen years, the number of patients on the books in Ontario provincial asylums dropped by about 75%, whereas the rates of admissions doubled, and those of discharges almost tripled (table 3.1). The proportion of readmissions doubled to form two-thirds of all admissions (Woogh et al, 1977). Provincial laws were altered to enable cost-sharing arrangements with the federal government to be made. The general hospital was encouraged to develop psychiatric service units, and provincial hospital patients could be transferred to community residential or nursing homes on a cost-sharing basis. In addition, provincial ministries other than Health would share the burden of costs in certain rehabilitation programs (Lemieux, 1977). In a very short time, the level of psychiatric care-giving outside the asylum in psychiatric units of general hospitals and in community-based mental health care has increased dramatically (table 3.2).

Table 3.2. Patient census at psychiatric units of general hospitals and community mental health facilities, Province of Ontario, 1965–1976. (Sources: Ontario Ministry of Health *Hospital Statistics*, 1974, and Ontario Ministry of Health unpublished data.)

Year	Psychiatric units			Community mental health facilities		
	admissions	discharges	'on books'	admissions	discharges	'on books'
1965	8815	8458	617	17319	16421	10042
1970	18914	18820	1118	37537	33729	28156
1974	26794	26702	1340	49417	47660	53637
1976	33299	32212	1789	data unavailable		

3.8 Postscript

There seems little doubt that the 'community' in Ontario, and elsewhere, was unprepared for the impact of the community mental health movement. Until recently, there have been no comprehensive bylaws in Ontario governing the various types of treatment facilities for handicapped groups. As these services have expanded, so has the confusion over proper definitions for these community-based facilities. In Toronto in 1977, for example, there were definitions for boys' homes, girls' homes, children's homes, children's shelters, boarding or lodging homes, foster homes, and haven or refuge homes. Each had different zoning restrictions. An attempt to locate a facility not covered by these definitions in a residential neighbourhood (such as an outpatient clinic) required a special hearing of the Ontario Municipal Board (the provincial 'court' of planning appeals). Such a hearing would inevitably be attended by those in opposition to the facility, who have frequently been successful in blocking neighbourhood access for mental health facilities. As a consequence, less vocal neighbourhoods have found themselves with a geographical concentration of facilities for various handicapped groups, including the mentally ill.

Recent attempts to establish 'fair share' zoning in major Ontario cities (Toronto, Hamilton) could facilitate the establishment of community mental health facilities, and clarify the moral obligation of all communities to care for their mentally ill. Such a policy, however, assumes that these facilities can be successfully integrated into different kinds of communities. It is not at all clear that this is the case. Moreover, the impact of this legislation on public response to the continuing trend toward community-based mental health care is uncertain.

Beliefs about mental illness and mental patients

Public beliefs about mental illness and the mentally ill are integrally linked with the social history of the asylum discussed in the previous chapter. For our purposes, they are of direct relevance because of their central role in the model of individual response to neighbourhood mental health facilities presented in chapter 2. Professional and public beliefs about the mentally ill have been the focus of considerable research in the fields of social psychology and psychiatry. Although no previous studies have to our knowledge examined the link between these beliefs and reactions to facilities for the mentally ill, the existing literature is important in the context of the present study both from a theoretical and from a methodological standpoint. In theoretical terms, these previous studies indicate the origin and covariates of beliefs about the mentally ill, that is, the external variables which influence belief formation. In terms of methodology, the existing literature reports the development of several different scales for measuring beliefs. Within this literature the term 'attitudes' is frequently applied to the concept which we prefer to label 'beliefs'. In this chapter we will conform with the literature and use the terms interchangeably. In subsequent chapters we shall maintain the distinction between them consistent with the structure of our model.

A comprehensive literature review is not attempted in this chapter. This would be redundant given the excellent reviews that already exist (see Rabkin, 1972; 1974; 1975). Our primary concern is to distil from previous research the theoretical and methodological implications for testing our model. We therefore focus on three main issues: factors affecting the formation of public beliefs about the mentally ill, methods for measuring public beliefs, and the relationship between beliefs and behaviour.

4.1 Factors affecting public beliefs about the mentally ill
The literature on public beliefs about mental illness and the mentally ill centres on two main themes. The first has been to trace changes in beliefs over time as a function of changing philosophies about mental illness and as a response to deliberate efforts to educate the public about the mentally ill. The second theme has been to examine the factors leading to variations in beliefs among different population subgroups at any one point in time. The first theme is therefore essentially longitudinal in its focus whereas the second is cross-sectional. It is the second which is of primary concern for our purpose, but before turning to it, it is important to note the conclusions that have been reached about changes in beliefs within society as a whole.

Despite ongoing controversies within the literature, most commentators are agreed that the last twenty-five years has seen a significant increase in public knowledge about the mentally ill (Rabkin, 1975; Halpert, 1969). This is reflected in the virtual disappearance of formerly widely held myths such as insanity is God's punishment for sin. Equally, the improved ability of the public to label mental illness correctly from case descriptions, demonstrated in more recent studies, reflects an advance in the state of knowledge. Together with this increased knowledge has come a greater tolerance of the mentally ill, although opinion is divided about the degree to which public attitudes have softened. The emergence of a more favourable disposition has been linked to the general acceptance of the medical model of mental illness; this is based on the premise that mental illness is an illness like any other. Efforts to educate the public to achieve acceptance of the medical model are generally seen to have been successful. At the same time, reviewers are careful to distinguish between acceptance in principle and in practice. Rabkin (1975, page 452) points out that although people generally accept the medical model as the 'correct' thing to believe, they still tend to avoid close contact with someone who is or has been mentally ill. In Rabkin's words: "people know they should regard mental illness as an illness like any other, but their feelings are not regularly shaped by their cognitive awareness". This inconsistency between principle and practice lends support to the model of mental illness which has been developed from labelling theory (Scheff, 1966; 1967). This model emphasizes the importance of social groups as the creators of deviance by the construction and application of rules of appropriate conduct. An implication of this view is that social rejection of mental patients has accelerated in recent years because the advent of community-based mental health care has increased the likelihood of contact between those labelled mentally ill and the general public. Thus, the conclusion that the public today are more favourably disposed toward the mentally ill than twenty years ago has to be carefully qualified.

Regardless of changes in the general climate of public opinion about mental illness and the mentally ill, there is substantial evidence to show that, at any one point in time, beliefs and attitudes vary as a function of several factors. Broadly speaking these factors fall into three sets which Rabkin (1975) labels as: characteristics of patients and treatment situations, characteristics of individuals within the general public, and characteristics of the social context. We shall discuss each of these in turn.

4.1.1 Effects of patient characteristics and treatment situation on public beliefs

Rabkin (1975) distinguishes eight characteristics of patients which have been shown in previous research to affect public beliefs about the mentally ill. The first and probably best documented is the perceived unpredictability of the patient. The more unpredictable the patient's behaviour is perceived to be the greater the rejection and avoidance. The consistency of this relationship has led Nunnally (1961) to conclude that unpredictability is a cornerstone of public attitudes toward the mentally ill.

To some extent associated with degrees of unpredictability is accountability. Avoidance and rejection are more likely if individuals are seen as not accountable or responsible for their behaviour. As such, they are typically labelled 'sick' rather than 'immoral' (See, 1968).

The demographic and social characteristics of the patient also influence public beliefs and attitudes. In general, more negative attitudes are held toward patients who are male (Phillips, 1964. Linsky, 1970), of lower social status (Linsky, 1970; Goffman, 1961; Bord, 1971), and who lack social ties within the community (Linsky, 1970). The observable symptoms of mental illness are also important. Physical symptoms tend to be less negatively perceived than behavioural symptoms. Especially important is the extent to which violent acts are a manifestation of illness. Violence and rejection are strongly correlated (Rabkin, 1975). A more subtle factor is the mystification surrounding the patient's illness. Symptoms and behaviours which can be understood tend to be less threatening than those which remain incomprehensible. This relationship is in part linked to the influence of unpredictability. The effects of these different symptoms to a large extent can be summarized in terms of the degree of social visibility in deviant behaviour. In Rabkin's words: "In our culture it is less socially acceptable to behave in a disruptive, bizarre or troublesome fashion than to act withdrawn, detached or depressed" (1975, page 455).

Several characteristics of the treatment situation can also be identified as influencing public beliefs and attitudes. The work of Hirsch and Borowitz (1973) is particularly instructive. They suggest an ordering of treatment sites based on the degree of negative feeling they arouse. In order of decreasing negativism they are: state mental hospital, private mental hospital, hospitals with integrated psychiatric and medical beds, and, finally, rest homes and spas. As others have pointed out, this ordering probably better reflects the social status of the patient than the severity of the disorder (Klee et al, 1967); nevertheless, the perception in the public's mind cannot be ignored. The ordering implies that the increasing emphasis on community-based care may serve to engender more positive public attitudes, but such a simple inference ignores the effects of increased contact between the mentally ill and the public resulting from the greater use of community facilities. Hirsch and Borowitz also suggest that public attitudes toward the mentally ill vary according to the method and frequency of treatment they receive. Somatic therapies are viewed more negatively than verbal therapies because they are presumed to imply more severe disorders. Those receiving more frequent treatments are perceived to be more seriously ill and hence more threatening. These are often misperceptions and incorrect inferences, but again their influence cannot be disregarded. Finally, the type of therapist consulted can also affect public attitudes. Least stigma is attached to consultations with non-psychiatric personnel (Phillips, 1963).

In a related study on the hierarchy of public preferences toward different disability groups, Tringo (1970) found that the mentally ill were least acceptable to the survey respondents. Other unacceptable groups were alcoholics, the mentally retarded, and ex-convicts; at the opposite end of the spectrum, the most acceptable disabilities were predominantly related to physical problems such as arthritis. A more recent survey by the Longwoods Research Group (1980) in Ontario tended to suggest a shift in the preference hierarchy.   Respondents ranked the acceptability of group homes for different client groups as follows: senior citizens (most acceptable), physically handicapped, mentally retarded, psychiatric problems, emotionally disturbed teenagers, alcohol problems, problems with the law (least acceptable). Of course, the response pattern is compounded because the survey addressed specific problems of group homes. However, this also emphasizes the importance of the client–facility link, which is a major distinction in our study.

For convenience and clarity, the effects of these various patient and treatment situation characteristics have been enumerated separately. In actual fact they operate in combination, with the result that attitudes toward a particular patient or group of patients result from a synthesis of factors which may not necessarily be mutually consistent. The formation of an individual's beliefs and attitudes is made all the more complex when the effects of his or her own characteristics are taken into account and it is to these that we now turn.

4.1.2 Effects of personal characteristics on public beliefs

Beliefs about mental illness and the mentally ill have been related to various personal characteristics of respondents in social surveys. Although characteristics such as age, education, occupation, social class, race, and ethnicity are interrelated, attempts have been made to examine their separate effects.

A large body of research has centred on the attitudes of mental hospital employees toward mental patients (Rabkin, 1972). The general conclusion is that there is a strong relationship between occupational status in the mental health field and attitudes toward mental patients. Occupational status was seen to be largely shaped by age, education, and social class. Persons with lower occupational status were found to be more authoritarian and restrictive, those of higher status were generally more liberal and tolerant (Gilbert and Levinson, 1956; Cohen and Struening, 1963; 1964; 1965).

The measures developed in research with mental health workers have often been used in studies with the general public. These studies have shown similar relationships. Freeman (1961), MacLean (1969) and Woodward (1951) found that low age and high education level were related to more 'scientific' and 'enlightened' kinds of knowledge about mental illness. Clark and Binks (1966), Freeman (1961), MacLean (1969),

Ramsey and Seipp (1948a; 1948b), and Whatley (1959) all found increased age and lower education to be associated in varying degrees with more unsympathetic, rejecting, and socially distant attitudes toward the mentally ill. No significant relationship between the sex of the respondent and attitudes has been found. Farina et al (1973) did find that the sex of the respondent and of the ex-mental patient were important variables associated with the acceptance granted an ex-mental patient as a prospective co-worker. But this study did not examine all the combinations of the variables so no definite conclusion that females were more accepting than males can be made. Marked differences have been noted in the prevalence and severity of mental illness, and the type of treatment sought and received, according to socioeconomic status (Hollingshead and Redlich, 1958). There is also some evidence that public attitudes toward mental illness and the mentally ill vary according to socioeconomic status of the respondent.

Cumming and Cumming (1957), Hollingshead and Redlich (1958), Lemkau and Crocetti (1962) and Star (1955) had all noted that there appeared to be a tendency on the part of the lower status and poorly educated groups to deny pathological conditions and deviant behaviour as being mentally ill. Did this mean that their tolerance of this behaviour was greater? No definite conclusion has been made about the relationship between the ability to identify behaviour in case descriptions and rejection and acceptance when measured by social distance scales.

Dohrenwend and Chin-Shong (1967) examined data from their previous studies for a relationship between the identification of behaviour in case descriptions as 'mentally ill' and tolerance of that behaviour. Tolerance was evaluated by the type of treatment recommended for the individual described. Dohrenwend and Chin-Shong reasoned that higher status groups were more apt to regard deviant behaviour as manifestations of mental illness than lower status groups. Through the process of formal education the higher status groups had been exposed to the psychiatric framework of symptoms and behaviour. They had also been exposed to and had accepted the humanistic, liberal message of the mental health profession. The lower status groups' living conditions and educational experiences had made them less receptive to the liberal, humanistic orientation and less knowledgeable of the psychiatric viewpoint and its application.

When lower status groups viewed behaviour as severely deviant or mentally ill, they tended to make the drastic recommendation of commitment to a mental hospital much more frequently than higher status groups. Dohrenwend and Chin-Shong felt that the lower status group definition of mental illness involved aggressive and antisocial behaviour. For the same behaviour (paranoid schizophrenia), higher status groups more often recommended outpatient treatment. Dohrenwend and Chin-Shong concluded that lower status groups were actually more intolerant of

serious mental illness than the higher status groups.   Bord (1971) questioned
the assumption that those exposed to this 'enlightened' perspective, the
higher status groups, showed any greater tolerance.   He felt that, although
expressed attitudes among the higher status group would continue to be
enlightened, reactions would remain largely rejecting in nature.

It is difficult to isolate attitudes toward mental illness that are directly
attributable to race or ethnic characteristics.   Social status, education, and
occupational level are all variables that are interrelated and directly related
to racial and ethnic membership.   Some studies have cited results which
indicate that blacks have expressed more traditional and less sympathetic
attitudes toward those labelled mentally ill.   Lemkau and Crocetti (1962)
reported that fewer blacks than whites expressed very favourable attitudes
toward psychiatric home care over hospitalization of mental patients.   This
association did not hold for the lowest education level.   There was no
attitudinal difference between the very poorly educated black and white
respondents.   Fournet (1967) conducted a study of several Louisiana
communities, and concluded that, compared to white respondents, blacks
were more restrictive and authoritarian toward the mentally ill and were
less likely to seek help from mental health professionals.   Rabkin (1974)
points out that it is very likely that Fournet's southern sample of blacks
occupied the lowest social position of any group studied.   The greater
degree of rejection by blacks could well be a result of minimal education
and very low status.   Ring and Chein's (1970) study of Cache Creek,
where the sample was predominantly black, upwardly mobile, and lower
middle class, indicates that black respondents were very similar to a
comparable sample of white respondents with regard to attitudes toward
mental illness and the mentally ill.   This supports the general conclusion
that race alone is not significantly associated with attitudes toward mental
illness.

4.1.3 Effects of social context on public beliefs
In terms of the effects of social context on public beliefs and attitudes
about the mentally ill, Rabkin (1975) identifies the availability of
psychiatric services in the community as particularly important.   The shift
in mental health care from institutions to community-based facilities has
meant that an increasingly large segment of the public are coming into
contact with discharged mental patients and have the opportunity to
witness, albeit from the outside, the operation of psychiatric facilities.
The advent of community-based care should therefore reduce the remote-
ness and isolation which for so long has characterized the history of
mental health care (see chapter 3).   The potentially increased familiarity
and contact with the mentally ill can have both positive and negative
effects on public attitudes.

The possibility provided by community facilities for the public to
observe ex-patients functioning within a normal environment should, in

principle at least, encourage greater public acceptance. We previously cited
the work of Hirsch and Borowitz which shows that treatment settings are
ordered in the public's mind in terms of the negative feelings they arouse.
An implication of their findings is that community facilities in general
arouse the least negative reactions. But this optimistic appraisal of the
potential influence of community-based care has to be tempered by recent
evidence from areas which have launched major deinstitutionalization
programs.

Rabkin (1975) cites California and New York as examples of cities where
rapid shifts to community-based care have had detrimental effects. The
basic problem was that communities were required to absorb too many
discharged patients too soon, with the result that inadequate provision had
been made in terms of support services and housing. In both instances,
the problem became a very contentious political issue leading in the
California case to a reversal of previous policy prior to the 1973 guber-
natorial elections, and to the suspension of the phasing-out of state
hospitals. Similar, if less extreme, situations have occurred in many other
North American cities. In Toronto, our study area, adverse reactions to
ex-mental patients have arisen because of their overconcentration in
certain parts of the city. It seems clear that there exists a saturation (or
'tipping') point in terms of the number of ex-patients that a community
can absorb, and that once this is exceeded the potentially positive effects
of community-based care on public attitudes will evaporate. In fact, there
may well be a reverse trend and public attitudes may harden. As a result,
the desire to exclude the mentally ill is perpetuated and we observe the
transition which Aviram and Segal (1973) have described from 'back
wards' to 'back alleys'. From a planning perspective, the problem lies in
accurately defining this saturation point and, at the same time, achieving
an equitable distribution of ex-patients such that no one community is
required to absorb more than can be reasonably expected. But political
obstacles arise and these can prevent the achievement of planning
objectives, with the result that the practice of exclusion is perpetuated and
there is very little evidence of greater public acceptance of the mentally ill.

Clearly these are issues and concerns which are central to our research
objectives, and we will return to them at various points as we discuss the
results and conclusions of our empirical work. For present purposes, it is
sufficient to observe that the social context within which the public
encounters the mentally ill can have a significant influence on beliefs and
attitudes.

4.1.4 Summary
We have seen that an amalgam of factors influence the formation of public
beliefs and attitudes about the mentally ill. Broadly, these divide into
personal and situational characteristics. Although it can be argued that
beliefs are fundamentally rooted in the individual psyche and reflect

personality, demographic, and social influences, they are also shaped by the context within which the individual encounters the mentally ill. In this latter respect, the characteristics of the patient, treatment situation, and general social context within which mental health care is provided are all important. Given the complex interaction between these different factors, isolating the effects of any single variable is very difficult, and it is not clear that previous research has been successful in doing so. There are additional remaining ambiguities which complicate the interpretation of existing findings. Perhaps primary amongst these is the label used to identify the mentally ill in opinion surveys. Our overview has indicated that a wide variety of labels has been used, including the 'mentally ill', 'mental patient', 'ex-mental patient', and 'ex-psychiatric patient'. It is far from clear what effect the use of different labels has on reported beliefs and attitudes, but, as Sarbin and Mancuso (1972) point out, it seems reasonable to expect a difference in response to those labelled as currently ill and those described as formerly ill. Because of this, caution is necessary in applying measurement procedures developed in an institutional context in studies of attitudes toward the mentally ill in the community.

4.2 Measurement of beliefs about the mentally ill

Previous studies contain a variety of instruments for measuring beliefs and attitudes about the mentally ill. They broadly fall into three groups: vignettes, social distance scales, and multiple item scales. The purpose of each method is different. The vignette method, originally developed by Star (1955), aimed to measure people's ability to identify mental illness. Social distance scales were introduced by Bogardus (1933) and modified for use in the mental health field by Whatley (1959). They are designed to measure the degree of acceptance that an individual will accord to a mentally ill person. Multiple item scales have the primary purpose of identifying and measuring the psychological dimensions corresponding to beliefs about the mentally ill. For the measurement of public beliefs, multiple item scales are the most appropriate and therefore must merit principal consideration in this section. Nevertheless, brief comment on the other two methods is justified.

Star's original vignettes consist of six case descriptions presented in everyday language. Respondents are asked which of the six they consider descriptive of someone who is mentally ill. The cases include a neurotic depressive, a paranoid schizophrenic, a simple schizophrenic, an alcoholic, a juvenile conduct disorder, and a phobic-compulsive neurotic. Comparison of results over time from different studies can reveal how public conceptions of what constitutes mental illness have changed. Equally, comparison across groups at one point in time can show how recognition of mental illness varies within the population. The problem with the vignettes is that the information so derived in itself provides no direct measure of how favourably or unfavourably the mentally ill are perceived.

Partly for this reason, they have often been used in conjunction with other methods such as social distance scales. Work in progress in Philadelphia (Rutman et al, 1980) shows how the vignette approach can be applied to measure potential acceptance of the mentally ill and of mental health facilities in a community context. For the Philadelphia study, new case descriptions are being used in conjunction with social distance scales to define public acceptance of different types of mental illness described in terms of overt behavioural characteristics. In addition, simple vignettes have been constructed describing the characteristics of different community-based facilities, and respondents are asked to indicate their willingness to accept each one into their neighbourhood. These are promising developments, particularly because they have been designed for application in a community context, unlike most of the original instruments.

Social distance scales are very simple in concept. They consist of six to eight statements ordered on a continuum of social interaction. Respondents indicate their willingness or nonwillingness to interact with a hypothetical mental patient in each of the ways described by the statements. Whatley's hypothetical patients were labelled as: someone formerly hospitalized, someone with mental problems, and someone who sees a psychiatrist. As previously mentioned, social distance scales have been frequently used in conjunction with vignettes to determine the degree of acceptable interaction with patients presented as case descriptions. As Rabkin (1975, page 452) comments, the results from studies using social distance scales are open to wide interpretation since it is not clear "what amount of social distance contributes rejection and what proportion of a sample must choose the social distance that is established as rejecting". In principle, it would seem possible to calibrate a social distance scale in terms of acceptance/rejection if information on behavioural intention and/or actual behaviour toward the mentally ill was collected in conjunction with the scale data. Unfortunately, in previous studies there has been a general failure to correlate social distance measures (and other belief and attitude measures) with behavioural criteria. Their predictive value therefore remains uncertain.

Likert scaling has been the most popular method for developing multiple item scales, although there are also examples of semantic differential scales (Nunnally, 1961; Fracchia et al, 1976; Olmstead and Durham, 1976). The use of multiple items rather than dependence on a single item enhances scale reliability and validity because the contribution of error variance to measured scores is reduced. Likert scales consist of a set of statements, each of which taps a particular aspect of the underlying belief or attitude dimension. Respondents record their degree of agreement or disagreement with each statement on a five-point labelled scale ranging from 'strongly agree' to 'strongly disagree' with a 'neutral' midpoint. The overall scale score is normally calculated as the unweighted sum of the individual statement responses.

Gilbert and Levinson's 'custodial mental illness scale' (CMI) was the first Likert scale to be widely used for measuring beliefs about the mentally ill (Gilbert and Levinson, 1956). The scale represents a single belief dimension which distinguishes between custodial and humanistic views of the mentally ill. Rabkin (1975, page 438) summarizes this polarization as follows:

"The extreme custodial point of view holds that mental patients cannot ever be really cured, that they are potentially dangerous and need external controls; in general, it is associated with authoritarianism and is highly correlated with the California F Scale. Its converse, humanism, is related to a generally egalitarian orientation."

Doubts as to whether beliefs about the mentally ill could be contained within a single dimension prompted the development of the 'opinions about mental illness' scales (OMI) by Cohen and Struening (1962). The OMI scales were originally developed in a study of the attitudes of hospital personnel toward mental illness. The OMI comprises five Likert scales which were empirically derived from a factor analysis of a pool of one hundred opinion statements. The statement pool was compiled primarily on a rational basis to reflect a range of sentiments about mental illness and the mentally ill, but it also drew upon existing scales such as the CMI, the California F scale (Adorno et al, 1950) and Nunnally's (1957) multiple item scale. The five OMI scales were labelled as: *authoritarianism*, reflecting a view of the mentally ill as an inferior class requiring coercive handling; *benevolence*, a paternalistic, sympathetic view of patients, based on humanistic and religious principles; *mental hygiene ideology*, the medical model view of mental illness as an illness like any other; *social restrictiveness*, viewing the mentally ill as a threat to society; and *interpersonal etiology*, reflecting a belief that mental illness arises from stresses in interpersonal experiences. These scales are almost certainly inter-correlated to some extent. The observed intercorrelation has varied between the different studies using the OMI (Fracchia et al, 1972).

The OMI has been the most widely used and best validated set of scales. Several other instruments have been devised, the most significant of which (for our purposes) is the 'community mental health ideology' scale (CMHI). Devised by Baker and Schulberg (1967), the CMHI was designed specifically to measure the ideology underlying the community mental health movement. The scale is unidimensional and comprises thirty-eight opinion statements expressing five concepts of the basic ideology. It has been shown to discriminate effectively between groups known to be highly oriented to this ideology and random samples of mental health professionals.

As Rabkin (1975) points out, the purpose for which the OMI and similar multiple item scales have been used has varied depending on the sample population. Studies of public beliefs focus on the stigma and social rejection associated with mental patients, whereas studies involving mental health professionals and personnel emphasize ideological positions and beliefs about the origins, nature, and outcomes of mental illness.

Compared with other types of measures, multiple item scales seem best able to uncover the psychological dimensions underlying beliefs about the mentally ill. At the same time, existing scales appear deficient in two important respects for application in studies of community reaction to neighbourhood mental health facilities. First, with the exception of the CMHI, their development predates the community mental health movement. They therefore presume or imply institutionalized care, and their validity for studies conducted in the context of community-based facilities has to be questioned. Second, the existing scales were primarily developed and applied in a professional context. It is relevant, therefore, to consider possible revisions to ensure that the opinion statements are expressed in a manner which is accessible to the general public. Because of these deficiencies we found it necessary to devise a new set of scales for our study (see chapter 6).

4.3 Beliefs and behaviour

The controversy in the behavioural research literature surrounding the relationship between personal dispositions (such as beliefs and attitudes) and behaviour extends to the mental health field. Researchers have often made naive assumptions that beliefs and attitudes are simple determinants of overt behaviour (Rabkin, 1974). They have failed to recognize that the factors which influence several attitudinal responses are not necessarily the same social and situational variables which determine *actual* behaviour in *specific* circumstances. Studies of the relationship between attitudes and behaviour with respect to the mentally ill are therefore often guilty of the faults which Fishbein and Ajzen (1975) have identified as reasons for the weak and inconsistent empirical findings in the attitude–behaviour link.

There are relatively few studies in the mental health literature which specifically address the attitude–behaviour relationship, although there are many which consider it in an anecdotal fashion. Among the specifically designed studies, Cohen and Struening (1962), using the OMI scales, examined the relationship between the beliefs of hospital staff and behaviour toward the mentally ill. The length of stay of patients in hospital was used as a surrogate measure of staff behaviour. Patients in hospitals where staff members expressed the most authoritarian and restrictive attitudes remained fewer days in the community during the six-month period after admission than did patients in other hospitals. Although there is some question as to the reasons for patient discharge, a link between attitude and behaviour was inferred.

Ellsworth (1965) investigated whether the endorsement of specific attitudes by mental hospital staff was related to significant differences in staff behaviour as rated by the patients. Statements were taken from the OMI and other scales. The relationships between attitudes and behavioural ratings were not completely consistent. The strongest most consistent link with behaviour was for the attitude dimension labelled 'restrictive control'.

Staff endorsing this attitude were rated by patients as impatient, rigid, domineering, and inconsiderate. This finding together with that from the Cohen and Struening study indicates that the attitudinal dimension of restrictiveness may have the strongest link with behaviour.

Fischer (1971) examined the relationship between humanitarian–altruistic attitudes, beliefs about mental illness, and the behavioural intention of community college students to work as volunteers with mental hospital patients. Fischer found that there was a substantial correspondence between the measure of intended behaviour to volunteer and later performance. The largest, but not highly significant, correlation between attitude measures and intended behaviour was for the altruism variable. Beliefs about mental illness had little bearing on altruism and intended behaviour. Several factors could account for the failure to find a relationship between attitudes about mental illness and intended behaviour to volunteer. Fischer did not take into account competing needs, attitudes, and situational variables such as course load, academic standing, extra-curricular activity, and financial needs (Rabkin, 1974). Following Fishbein and Ajzen's (1972) argument, if attitudes toward volunteer work, a specific attitude, had been measured a relationship might have been found with the intended behaviour of volunteering to work with mental patients (Rabkin, 1974).

In terms of anecdotal findings, LaFave et al (1967) reported a study of two Canadian communities, Cloverdale and DeLis, with significantly different attitudes about mental illness. Cloverdale respondents held significantly more sophisticated and enlightened attitudes than those of DeLis. During the course of this study, information became available that was relevant to the relationship between attitudes and actual behaviour of the respondents. The researchers obtained data for all persons with the diagnosis of psychosis, psychoneurosis, and character disorder admitted to general hospitals and to the mental hospital which served the two towns. LaFave et al stated that "it might be concluded that although the overall rate of persons admitted to any hospital from the two towns is very similar there is a greater tendency for the mentally ill of DeLis to be admitted to 'general' hospitals rather than to the 'mental' hospital (LaFave et al, 1967, page 224). The researchers also became aware of a petition that had been circulated in Cloverdale, bearing one-third of the adult population's signatures. The petition was against the establishment of a halfway house for ex-mental patients previously from the area. The half-way house never opened. In contrast, the town of DeLis had supported the operation of three foster homes for ex-mental patients for approximately three years. LaFave felt that these occurrences point out the mistake of concluding direct relationships between attitudes expressed in an interview and questionnaire format and actual behaviour. The assumption cannot be made that tolerant behaviour toward the mentally ill will come from those expressing sophisticated attitudes about mental illness. DeLis residents who, in the survey, tended to deny mental illness and held less sophisticated attitudes, were less inclined to practice isolation through mental hospital-ization and insulation by preventing former mental patients access to halfway or foster home residence.

Considered overall, few studies have shown clear relationships between measures of beliefs or attitudes and behaviour toward the mentally ill. This seems especially true of those studies involving the general public and conducted in a community, rather than hospital, setting. As indicated earlier, part of the problem lies in methodological failings such as the lack of correspondence between attitude and behaviour measures. There are other difficulties, however, which are less easily overcome. Possibly the most important of those is the influence of social norms on verbal expressions of beliefs and attitudes. The prevailing climate of opinion within society determines which attitudes are socially acceptable and which are not, and there is a strong tendency for questionnaire respondents to conform to the norm, and to avoid expressing socially unacceptable opinions. The direction of this normative influence presently is away from authoritarian and restrictive views and toward more benevolent and sympathetic attitudes. The potential confounding effect of this sort of convergence to prevailing norms has led some researchers to doubt the values of questionnaire-based measures of attitudes and to recommend the use of unobtrusive methods when possible (Page, 1977). In principle, unobtrusive methods provide an attractive alternative to questionnaire methods, but in practice it is often very difficult to devise them, despite the imaginative guidelines in the literature (Webb et al, 1966). Perhaps more fruitful in the long term is to conduct more carefully designed studies, taking account of the factors identified by Fishbein and Ajzen (1975), and to include several different independent measures of attitudes rather than rely upon a single measure which may be too vulnerable to confounding influences.

4.4 Conclusions
Several important implications for our analysis of community responses to neighbourhood mental health facilities derive from the issues addressed in this chapter. The first concerns the *importance of beliefs* about the mentally ill for explaining public acceptance or rejection of mental patients and, by extension, of mental health facilities. As described in chapter 2, our theoretical model places considerable importance on these beliefs. There seems little doubt in the literature that beliefs and attitudes play a fundamental role in determining behavioural responses to the mentally ill. This conviction remains despite the equivocal results of studies linking beliefs and attitudes with behaviour. This lack of success is generally attributed to methodological problems rather than to the lack of a relation-ship between attitudes and behaviour. Although previous studies have not

specifically examined the link between beliefs about the mentally ill and reactions to mental health facilities, it seems reasonable to assume that public beliefs are potentially very important explanatory variables in this context also.

Besides providing general support for our model, the literature on attitudes toward the mentally ill identifies many *factors which influence belief and attitude formation* and which therefore have to be considered for inclusion as external variables in the model. The factors described in this chapter essentially correspond with the three subsets of external variables in the model, namely facility/user characteristics, personal characteristics, and neighbourhood characteristics. The structure of the model is, therefore, consistent with the evidence from previous research. This is not to imply that the relationships between the external variables and beliefs about the mentally ill are already fully understood. As other reviewers have noted (Rabkin, 1975), past studies are open to serious criticism because of methodological and analytical weaknesses, with the result that the separate and joint effects of particular variables on public beliefs and attitudes are, in general, poorly understood.

Not only is there a need for studies which are methodologically stronger. Past research has generally focussed on attitudes toward the mentally ill in an institutional setting. Given the advent and spread of community-based mental health care, there is a vital need for research which explicitly deals with public reactions to the mentally ill *in a community context*. This is particularly important because an obvious consequence of a policy of deinstitutionalization is to increase the likelihood of contact between the mentally ill and the general public. Rabkin (1977) recognizes that increased contact between the mentally ill and the general public may engender friction in neighbourhoods and she argues that "... if the force of public attitudes is not taken into account, the eventual outcome may be exacerbation of public fears accompanied by a retreat to custodial care and removal from the community" (pages 1 and 2). Public reactions to the mentally ill in the community require careful studies because they potentially affect the success of deinstitutionalized care in two important respects. From the perspective of mental patients, the attitudes of residents in neighbourhoods with mental health facilities are of primary importance in determining their social integration in the community (see Segal and Aviram, 1978). From the perspective of the planner and politician, residents' attitudes are important in anticipating potential conflict situations resulting from the location of facilities in residential neighbourhoods.

Two important implications follow from the need to conduct research which has a community focus. The first is the need to *develop belief scales* which are relevant in a community context. Although existing scales such as the OMI provide a very good foundation, they are not ideally suited to community studies because they assume institutionalized care. Substantial revisions of existing instruments are necessary to incorporate the ideas and attitudes associated with social psychiatry and community psychology. The second implication concerns the *choice of label* to apply to the mentally ill in the community. We pointed out earlier that a variety of labels has been used without any systematic assessment of their differential effects on responses. For studies of public reaction to the mentally ill in community-based care it is important that the label accurately reflects the type of patient or ex-patient that the public are likely to encounter in their neighbourhood.

A final major implication from existing research is the need in any future study to *link beliefs and attitudes about the mentally ill with behaviour*. As noted previously, this has not been emphasized in earlier work, with the result that uncertainties remain about the attitudes–behaviour link and the factors affecting it. In chapter 2 we indicated that our ultimate objective is to explain and predict behavioural responses in terms of facility acceptance and rejection. The links between beliefs, attitudes, and behaviour are therefore fundamental to our theoretical model.

In sum, these various implications of previous research on beliefs and attitudes toward the mentally ill have helped to shape our own study of community response to neighbourhood mental health facilities. We find support for the basic structure of our model which emphasizes the importance of beliefs and attitudes as the antecedents of behaviour. Equally, the external variables affecting belief formation included in the model generally correspond to those identified in existing work. We recognize the need to develop new belief and attitude scales relevant to public opinions about the mentally ill in community-based care. Finally, we concur with the need expressed by other reviewers to investigate the behavioural correlates of public beliefs and attitudes.

Part 3: Research design

5 Toronto study design

We now shift attention from the theoretical and contextual basis of our analysis of community response to mental health facilities to the details of the Toronto study. To fulfill our empirical objectives, data were required from primary and secondary sources. Social survey data from a representative sample of Toronto area residents were needed to analyze nonuser reactions to facilities based on the theoretical model outlined in chapter 2. The remaining data requirements were met from secondary sources including census and land-use reports. In addition, real estate records provided data for a separate test of the effects of mental health facility locations on property values. In this chapter, we first briefly describe the data requirements for the study, and then outline the design of the questionnaire survey with reference to two main topics: sample selection and questionnaire development.

5.1 Data requirements for the Toronto study

The data requirements for the Toronto study were primarily determined by the theoretical model described in chapter 2. The model includes variables measured at two levels: the individual and the neighbourhood. The individual-level variables comprise personal characteristics (socio-economic status, demographic measures, personality variables, and past experience with mental illness and the mentally ill), beliefs, attitudes, behavioural intentions, and behaviour. The neighbourhood-level variables fall into two groups: mental health facility and user characteristics and neighbourhood physical and social structure.

A major questionnaire survey of a sample of Metropolitan Toronto residents provided the only feasible method of collecting the individual-level data. The potential importance of socioeconomic status and related variables on individual response to facilities led to the selection of a stratified random sample design for the survey with one of the two stratification criteria being socioeconomic status. The neighbourhood-level data were obtained from secondary sources. Information on the locations and service characteristics of mental health facilities in Metropolitan Toronto was obtained from a variety of agencies including psychiatric hospitals and community service groups. This information was fundamental to the sample design, since the sampling units (census enumeration areas) were selected on the basis of the presence or absence of facilities. Data on the physical and social structure of Toronto neighbourhoods were obtained from land-use reports compiled by the Metropolitan Toronto planning department. Neighbourhood considerations also entered into the sample design. We anticipated variations in reactions to facilities between city and suburban neighbourhoods, and for this reason a simple city–suburb distinction was used as the second stratification criterion for sample selection.

As part of our second major empirical objective, to determine the neighbourhood impacts of mental health facilities, we wanted to examine whether the location of facilities had had any measurable effect on property values. As indicated in chapter 2, fears of falling property values are frequently cited as a basis for opposition to facilities and our concern was to determine whether there are any empirical grounds for such fears. Real estate records, made available by the Toronto Real Estate Board were the source of data for this analysis. Full details of the data-collection procedures are given in chapter 9 which describes the results of the property value analysis and therefore no more attention is paid to them in this chapter.

5.2 Design of the questionnaire survey

5.2.1 Sample design and selection [1]

A rigorous test of the theoretical model required data from a sample representative of the Metropolitan Toronto population. A probability-based sample was therefore necessary, but a simple random sample of area residents was neither an efficient nor an effective design for our purposes. The major reason for this stems from the importance of neighbourhood-based characteristics, which argues for the use of areal sampling units. A multistage cluster sample was selected as the most cost-effective design, comprising three stages: neighbourhood selection, household selection within neighbourhoods, and respondent selection within households. Two multistage samples were drawn, one from areas with existing mental health facilities and one from areas without them. The rationale for this was to permit a comparison of the effects of facilities on local neighbourhoods as *experienced* by people living in areas with facilities, and as *expected* by people in areas without facilities. The two samples will be discussed separately beginning with the sample from areas without facilities.

Selection of the *without facilities sample* required the identification of existing facility locations so that areas with facilities could be excluded from the sampling frame. Also required was a definition of an appropriate areal sampling unit. A list of facility locations was compiled from various sources including psychiatric hospitals and community service groups. The list includes four main facility types: residential group homes and boarding homes, outpatient clinics (excluding any attached to psychiatric or general hospitals), centres providing social/therapeutic programs, and centres for vocational training. Identification of residential care facilities and especially commercial boarding homes was the most difficult, and it is quite possible that some facilities were missed because they do not appear on any existing records. Our search yielded a total of eighty-four facilities located in residential neighbourhoods within Metropolitan Toronto (table 5.1 and figure 5.1).

[1] The Survey Research Centre at York University, Toronto, had full responsibility for sample selection and data collection.

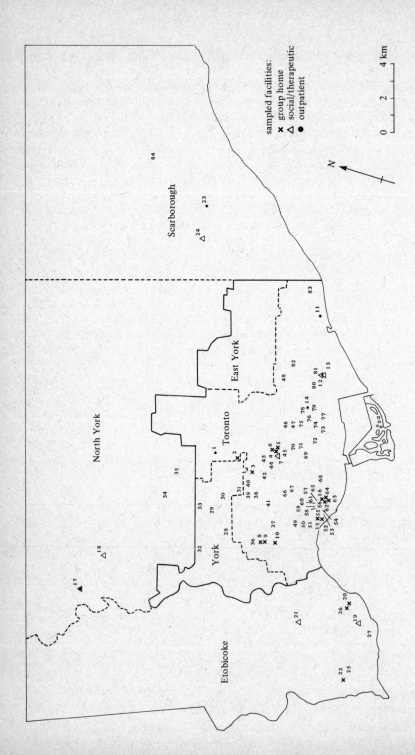

Figure 5.1. Distribution of community mental health facilities in Metropolitan Toronto in the city (City of Toronto and Boroughs of York and East York) and suburban (Boroughs of North York, Scarborough, and Etobicoke) zones.

The census enumeration area (CEA) was chosen as the areal sampling unit for the first stage of the sample design. Based on the 1971 census, there are 4836 CEAs in the Toronto census metropolitan area which in 1971 comprised 774000 households. There are, therefore, an average of 160 households per CEA. In areal terms, the size of CEAs varies considerably depending upon population density, with inner-city CEAs in general being much smaller than those in the suburbs. Although the CEA may not correspond well with traditional concepts of neighbourhood, it has two important advantages as a sampling unit. First, the CEA is sufficiently small that within-area variations in household characteristics are generally small thereby reducing the sampling error introduced by a cluster design. Second, data on household characteristics are available for each CEA, which facilitates the allocation of areas within any stratified design. In addition, the problem of the noncorrespondence of the CEA and larger neighbourhood units can be, at least partially, overcome by the aggregation of constituent CEAs for purposes of neighbourhood-level analyses.

The sampling frame for the without facilities sample therefore comprised all CEAs within the Toronto census metropolitan area with the exception of those CEAs containing one or more of the eighty-four existing facility locations. Two stratification criteria were used: socioeconomic status

Table 5.1. Distribution of known mental health facilities in Metropolitan Toronto[a] in city and suburban locations.

Facility type	Social status of location			Totals
	high	medium	low	
City[b]				
Group home	4	16	23	43
Social/therapeutic	3	5	6	14
Vocational	2	0	7	9
Outpatient	0	1	3	4
Subtotal	9	22	39	70
Suburbs[c]				
Group home	0	2	2	4
Social/therapeutic	1	1	3	5
Vocational	0	2	0	2
Outpatient	0	0	3	3
Subtotal	1	5	8	14
Overall total	10	27	47	84

[a] Excludes psychiatric hospitals and psychiatric units in general hospitals.
[b] Includes City of Toronto; Boroughs of York and East York.
[c] Includes Boroughs of North York, Scarborough, and Etobicoke.

(three levels: low, medium, and high) and geographic zone (two levels: city and suburb). CEAs were classified by socioeconomic status by means of a socioeconomic index devised by Greer-Wootten and Patel (1976). CEAs were ranked in ascending order on the index and the $33\frac{1}{3}$ and $66\frac{2}{3}$ percentiles were used as class boundaries. The two geographic zones (figure 5.1) were defined as follows:

city   the City of Toronto and the Boroughs of York and East York;
suburb   the Boroughs of North York, Scarborough, and Etobicoke.

CEAs were randomly selected within each of the six cells of the design. Six CEAs were selected in each of the low and high status cells and twelve in the middle status cells. The main reason for the higher sampling rate for the middle status areas was to permit a reliable analysis of tenure effects on reactions to facilities.

The selection of households involved listing all addresses within each of the forty-eight CEAs chosen in the first stage of sampling. From these listings 1031 households were randomly selected by means of a pre-determined selection ratio based on the household count for each CEA and on the desired number of households per CEA. The size of the selected sample (table 5.2) of 1031 households compared with the target of 720 reflects an expected completion rate of 66%.

The selection of respondents within households was carried out in the field by the interviewers. The sample design required that one eligible person (that is, permanent member of the household over eighteen years of age) be selected from each household. This involved listing all eligible persons in a household and then randomly selecting one person as the designated respondent. As many as five callbacks were made to reach a selected respondent.

The selection of respondents in *areas with facilities* also involved a multistage procedure. The initial sampling frame comprised CEAs containing one or more of the eighty-four neighbourhood-based mental health facilities. These CEAs were classified according to the same two stratification criteria used in the without facilities sample. Selection of CEAs within the six strata was purposive rather than random for two

Table 5.2. Household selection by strata: areas without facilities.

Geographic zone	Socioeconomic status[a]			Total
	low	middle	high	
City	118 (90)	253 (180)	129 (90)	500 (360)
Suburb	125 (90)	257 (180)	149 (90)	531 (360)
Total	243 (180)	510 (360)	278 (180)	1031 (720)

[a] Target sample in parentheses.

reasons. First, the total number of CEAs with facilities from which to draw a sample was small, hence greatly reducing the need for random selection to ensure representativeness. Second, it was considered more important that the CEAs be selected with reference to the type of facility located in them rather than on a purely random basis. Random selection would almost certainly have resulted in a failure to have areas with different types of facility represented in each of the sample strata. Twenty-one CEAs were therefore purposely selected, four in each cell except the high status suburban stratum for which there was only one eligible CEA. The four CEAs in the other five strata were selected such that two contained a residential care facility (that is, group home or boarding home) and two a nonresidential facility (that is, outpatient clinic or social/therapeutic centre). This selection procedure allowed comparison of reactions to the two most basic facility types: residential and non-residential.

The second and third stages of selection followed the same randomised procedures used for the sampling of areas without facilities. The allocation of households by strata (table 5.3) shows a total of 579 selected households compared with a target of 360, again reflecting an expected completion rate of 66%.

Table 5.3. Household selection by strata: areas with facilities.

Geographic zone	Socioeconomic status[a]			Total
	low	middle	high	
City	78 (60)	83 (60)	136 (60)	297 (180)
Suburb	97 (60)	103 (60)	82 (60)	282 (180)
Total	175 (120)	186 (120)	218 (120)	579 (360)

[a] Target sample in parentheses.

5.2.2 Sample evaluation

Data collection commenced in June 1978 and was completed in October 1978. Because of high refusal rates and absentee problems during the summer months of July and August, the anticipated completion rate of 66% was not achieved. Consequently, 546 supplementary households were selected from the same CEAs included in the original sample allocation (table 5.4). The breakdown of completions by strata for both samples (table 5.5) compared with the target allocation, shows that for the 'without facilities' sample the target was achieved for four of the six strata, the two exceptions being the low class and middle class cells in the city zone. This reflects the lower response rate typically encountered in lower class neighbourhoods. For the 'with facilities' sample, again the target was met for four strata. In this case a deficit occurred in the middle class city cell and high class suburban cell. The latter is explained by the restriction in that stratum to only one eligible CEA for household and respondent selection. Given that restriction, the number of completions (50) is surprisingly high. All households were contacted and so resampling in that cell was not possible.

A check was made on the effectiveness of the socioeconomic status stratification. The occupational data collected in the questionnaire was used in an analysis of variance to test for significant differences between the sample strata in occupational status [based on the Blishen scale (Blishen and McRoberts, 1976)]. The results showed a highly significant difference in the expected direction with the high status stratum having the highest mean occupational status scores and the low status stratum the lowest.

Table 5.4. Resample allocation for inner-city and suburban zones.

Social status	Without facilities		With facilities	
	CEA allocation	sample allocation	CEA allocation	sample allocation
Inner City				
Low	4	36	4	38
Medium	6	66	4	42
High	4	40	4	67
Suburb				
Low	4	42	4	49
Medium	6	63	4	51
High	4	52	–[a]	–
Total	28	299	20	247

[a] Enumeration area was exhausted.

Table 5.5. Number of interview completions by strata, both samples.

Geographical zone	Social status[a]			Totals
	low	middle	high	
Without facilities sample				
City	74 (90)	146 (180)	93 (90)	313 (360)
Suburb	95 (90)	180 (180)	114 (90)	389 (360)
Total	169 (180)	326 (360)	207 (180)	702 (720)
With facilities sample				
City	61 (60)	55 (60)	77 (60)	193 (180)
Suburb	67 (60)	78 (60)	50 (60)	195 (180)
Total	128 (120)	133 (120)	127 (120)	388 (360)

[a] Target sample in parentheses.

Table 5.6. Summary of field statistics.

Statistic	Selected households	Multiple households	Total households	Ineligible households[a]	Base	Completions	Ill/aged	Language problems	Refusals	Absent	Other
Original sample											
Count	1610	20	1630	75	1555	811	29	130	388	188	9
Completion rate (%)			100·0	4·5	95·5	49·8	1·8	8·0	23·8	11·5	0·6
Response rate (%)					100·0	52·1	1·9	8·4	24·9	12·1	0·6
Resample											
Count	546	8	544	14	540	279	11	40	107	94	9
Completion rate (%)			100·0	2·5	97·5	50·4	2·0	7·2	19·3	17·0	1·6
Response rate (%)					100·0	51·7	2·0	7·4	19·8	17·4	1·7
Total sample											
Count	2156	28	2184	89	2095	1090	40	170	495	282	18
Completion rate (%)			100·0	4·1	95·9	49·9	1·8	7·8	22·7	12·9	0·8
Response rate (%)					100·0	52·0	1·9	8·1	23·6	13·5	0·9

[a] Includes dead and vacant addresses.

The final set of field statistics (table 5.6) show that total completions numbered 1090 which represents a completion rate of $49 \cdot 9\%$ and a response rate of 52%, substantially lower than the expected rate of 66%. The discrepancy can be explained largely by the timing of the field work which coincided with the peak vacation months of July and August. The refusal rate of $23 \cdot 6\%$ for the total sample is somewhat higher than normally expected, again reflecting more reluctance on the part of the general public to participate in surveys during the summer months. The remaining $24 \cdot 4\%$ of the nonresponse rate is accounted for by one of four factors: respondents too ill or aged to complete the questionnaire (2%), respondents with language difficulties outside the expertise of the interviewing team (8%), absentee respondents after full quota of callbacks (13%), and respondents whose questionnaires were too incomplete to be of any use (1%). The relatively high nonresponse and refusal rates undoubtedly introduce a self-selection bias in the final sample of 1090. Identifiable biases include the selective exclusion of ethnic minorities whose first language was not one spoken by one of the interviewers (there were interviewers fluent in Italian, Portuguese, French, and Greek, as well as English). Given the timing of the data collection, people taking vacations in July and August were more likely to have been excluded. Whether these and other possible sources of bias are systematically related to reactions to the mentally ill and mental health facilities is unknown. It is important to note, however, that the survey was not introduced as a study of attitudes to the mentally ill and hence the refusal rate cannot be explained in terms of a reluctance to answer questions on this subject. There is, therefore, no strong evidence to suggest that the data obtained are seriously distorted or unrepresentative of the views of Metropolitan Toronto residents.

In summary, both samples were selected by means of a multistage cluster design. From CEAs without mental health facilities, a stratified random sample was drawn with the completed interviews closely approximating the target figures. From CEAs with facilities, respondent households were randomly selected within purposively chosen CEAs, again allocated within a stratified sample design. Completions also closely approximate target figures for this sample. The relatively low response rates for the total sample introduces the possibility of sample bias, but this is not seen seriously to distort the representativeness of the survey data.

5.2.3 Questionnaire design
In common with many questionnaire surveys the instrument designed for this study had a basic 'funnel' structure proceeding from general to specific questions [2]. The purpose of this approach is to introduce general contextual questions in the early part of the survey which often serve to

[2] Copies of the questionnaire may be obtained by writing to the authors at the Department of Geography, McMaster University, Hamilton, Ontario, Canada L8S 4K1.

place the more specific later questions in a clearer perspective. In addition, the 'funnel' structure avoids prompting the respondent to answer in a particular way; this may result if very specific structured questions are presented from the beginning. The use of general and more open-ended questions at the beginning also has the advantage of facilitating rapport between interviewer and respondent.

Given these considerations, the questionnaire was introduced as seeking information on "your feelings about various community services". Specific mention of mental health services was deliberately avoided to minimize the initial prompting given to the respondent and to provide an appropriate lead into the first few questions which dealt with general opinions about community services in residential neighbourhoods.

Following these, questions were asked to determine awareness of community mental health facilities in Toronto and the neighbourhood. Responses to these questions on awareness of a facility in the neighbourhood determined whether or not certain later questions were asked. It was therefore especially vital that the definition of a 'community mental health facility' be made as unambiguous as possible. Clarity in definition was also very important because the same label was to be used in several other subsequent questions. To this end a standard definition was read to each respondent emphasizing the range of facilities embraced by the label and their local, small-scale characteristics. The definition read as follows:

"Community mental health facilities include outpatient clinics, drop-in centres, and group homes which are situated in residential neighbourhoods and serve the local community. Mental health facilities which are part of a major hospital are *not* included."

The questions on awareness were followed by an open-ended question to determine the perceived or experienced effects of a community mental health facility on the neighbourhood. It was important to ask this question at this early stage since the content of subsequent questions would almost inevitably have affected the responses given.

The next section of the questionnaire elicited beliefs about mental illness and the mentally ill. It is probably a moot point whether these beliefs are better elicited before or after the questions on specific reactions to mental health facilities. It is not obvious which, if either, set of questions is the more likely to have a contaminating effect on the other. The belief questions comprised forty Likert statements representing four underlying dimensions derived from previous research on attitudes toward the mentally ill. It was vital that response to the belief statements be made with reference to a standard definition of the mentally ill. For the purposes of the study, the mentally ill were defined as "people needing treatment for mental disorders, but who are capable of independent living outside a hospital". This definition was read to respondents and it was made clear that the mentally retarded were excluded from this definition.

Beliefs about mental illness and the mentally ill were measured on four scales, three of which—authoritarianism, benevolence, and social restrictiveness—were originally developed by Cohen and Struening (1962), and the fourth—community mental health ideology—was developed by Baker and Schulberg (1967). The scales used in this study are major modifications of the originals. The modifications had three purposes: first, to make the belief statements relevant to community-based mental health care; second, to express the statements in a way immediately understandable by the general public (the original scales were developed and applied primarily in the context of professional psychiatry); third, to limit the number of statements for each scale within the constraints imposed by the projected length and duration of the entire questionnaire (twenty-five to thirty minutes). To these ends, each of the four scales is represented by ten statements, some of which are taken verbatim from the original scales. In writing new statements, the aim was to leave the underlying concept of the scale unchanged. The immediate check on this is in terms of the correlations between the original and new statements for each scale as reflected in the scale reliability coefficients reported in the next chapter.

Five of the ten statements on each scale expressed a positive sentiment with reference to the underlying concept and the other five were negatively worded. For example, for the authoritarianism scale, five statements expressed a proauthoritarian sentiment and five were antiauthoritarian. The response format for each statement was the standard Likert five-point labelled scale: strongly agree/agree/neutral/disagree/strongly disagree. The statements were sequenced in ten sets of four, and within each set the statements were ordered by scale: authoritarianism, benevolence, social restrictiveness, and community mental health ideology. The aim of this sequencing was to minimize possibilities of response set bias. Statements were self-administered except for respondents who were illiterate or for other reasons (for example, sight problem) had difficulty in reading. The procedure followed was for the interviewer to hand the questionnaire to the respondent after first reading the definition of the mentally ill as previously described. Full details of scale development are reported in the next chapter.

The next several questions were designed to elicit structured responses to community mental health facilities. The sequencing of these questions was in no sense arbitrary. Respondents were first asked to indicate their general perceptions of a community mental health facility by checking those adjectives from an alphabetical list which they associated with the term 'community mental health facility'. The earlier definition of the term was repeated to ensure standardization of responses. The same seventy-eight-item adjective check list was used in the following question to elicit perceptions of the local neighbourhood. The check list was selected in preference to other possible methods of measuring perceptions because of its flexibility, use of everyday language, ease of administration, and the minimum constraints imposed on responses. The initial pool of adjectives were drawn from Craik's (1971) *Environmental Adjective Check List* and subsequently reduced in number to yield an instrument of more manageable length containing only adjectives judged on an a priori basis to be immediately relevant to the stimuli of interest. The final list of seventy-eight adjectives represents six underlying a priori scales labelled: activity, evaluation, safety, integration, design, predictability. The following chapter discusses the development and testing of these scales in detail.

Consistent with the rationale of moving from more general to more specific questions, respondents were next asked to rate the impacts they perceived a community mental health facility would have (or has had in the case of respondents aware of a facility in their neighbourhood) on their neighbourhood. Twelve seven-point semantic differential scales devised from related studies (Gingell et al, 1975) were the basis for the ratings. The impact scales included tangible effects, such as changes in traffic volume and noise levels, and those less tangible effects such as changes in neighbourhood quality and residential character. The seven scale points were numbered 1 to 7 with only two poles labelled and the respondent circled the number best describing his perceptions of expected impact (if unaware of a facility in the neighbourhood) or experienced impact (if aware). For analytical purposes each scale can be treated separately. In addition, composite scales based on the total set or subsets of scales can be defined.

Following the impact ratings, a measure of overall attitude toward community health mental facilities was obtained. Respondents rated the desirability of a facility being located within three distances of their home: seven to twelve blocks, two to six blocks, and within one block. A nine-point labelled category scale was used ranging from 'extremely desirable' to 'extremely undesirable' with a neutral midpoint. The same scale had been used successfully in an earlier related study (Gingell et al, 1975). The three distance zones were used to provide one measure of the extent of the externality field of community mental health facilities. The distance zones were defined to separate reactions to a location at close proximity, one in an intermediate range, and one relatively distant from home. The breakpoint between one and two blocks is viewed as critical, that between six and seven blocks is probably more arbitrary. The use of a more detailed distance breakdown would have lengthened the questionnaire with little if any information being gained.

The desirability ratings were the basis for the next question which requested information on intended actions with respect to each facility location rated to some degree undesirable. Respondents were then asked if they had actually taken any of these actions to oppose a facility location. The focus on action taken in opposition to facilities reflects the project objectives of seeking to understand the basis and consequences of opposition. This is not to deny the possibility of actions supporting the location of community mental health facilities in residential neighbourhoods.

The next set of questions was dependent upon the respondent's awareness of a mental health facility in their neighbourhood. Those unaware were asked a single question about their anticipated change in attitude or behaviour if a mental health facility were to open in their neighbourhood. Those aware were asked a series of questions to determine their reaction to the existing facility.

The last question related to facilities was asked of all respondents and was open-ended, inviting suggestions about how best to fit mental health facilities into residential neighbourhoods.

As in many other questionnaires, the final set of questions elicited various demographic and socioeconomic indicators. These are generally best asked last because the rapport established between interviewer and respondent by this stage is normally sufficient to overcome any reluctance the respondent may feel in divulging this information. Unfortunately, constraints on the length of the questionnaire prevented the inclusion of questions to determine the personality characteristics of respondents. With this exception, however, the questionnaire provided all of the individual-level data needed to test the theoretical model.

5.2.4 Pretesting of the questionnaire

The final questionnaire as described in the previous two sections was the end result of careful pretesting. Three separate pretests were conducted. Two were carried out by the Survey Research Centre at York University who had responsibility for the data collection. One of these was in-house among a small group of employees ($N = 6$) conducted in March 1978. The second was a field pretest ($N = 54$) in various areas of Metropolitan Toronto carried out in April 1978 and designed to match the conditions for the major survey. The third pretest was limited to the beliefs about mental illness scales and sampled students in the first-year undergraduate class in urban geography at McMaster University ($N = 321$). The aim in this case was to assess the reliability and validity of the belief statements, and this is discussed in the next chapter.

Major revisions resulted from each pretest. The in-house York pretest showed that the proposed questionnaire was too lengthy. Average time for completion was about forty minutes compared with the target of twenty-five minutes. The version of the questionnaire used included questions on reactions to two other facilities (a fire station and library) in addition to mental health facilities. Given the time constraints the fire station questions were dropped. This was made all the more necessary because of the desire to include the beliefs about the mentally ill scales which were not in the earliest version of the questionnaire.

The York field pretest indicated several problems necessitating further revisions. The average duration of the questionnaire was still ten to fifteen minutes above the target, requiring substantial deletions. The interviewers reported that respondents were confused by the inclusion of questions on mental health and library facilities within the same questionnaire given the lack of any obvious connection between the two. The interviewer's answer that the study purposely sought opinions about two very different types of facility did little to ease the confusion. The apparent confusion, together with the need to shorten the questionnaire, led to the decision to drop the library-related questions. In so doing, the remaining 'control' facility against which to compare reactions to mental health facilities was lost. This was not regarded as a serious loss because the opening questions elicited responses about community services in general prior to any mention of mental health facilities, and, as such, provided a basis against which to compare the subsequent facility-specific reactions. Deleting the library questions was certainly more defensible than dropping any of the mental health questions.

The field pretest also revealed the need for more precise definitions of key terms, specifically, 'the mentally ill' with respect to the belief statements and the 'community mental health facility' label used in several key questions. As a result the definitions were rewritten to remove the apparent ambiguities. The final definitions were given in the previous section. An additional wording problem was encountered in the instructions for completing the adjective check lists particularly with reference to a community health mental facility. The pretest instructions asked respondents to check adjectives which for them were 'descriptive' of a mental health facility. Since many respondents said they had never seen one they were unsure how to respond. It was clear, therefore, that the instructions had to be rephrased to elicit, as intended, the connotations invoked by the term rather than a realistic description, which many respondents thought was required. To this end the wording of the instructions was changed to read "... put an x beside each (word) you *associate* with the term community mental health facility". Following this, the definition of the term was repeated.

5.3 Land-use and census data
In addition to the individual-level data obtained by the questionnaire, information concerning neighbourhood land-use mix and social structure was required to test the model of individual responses to mental health facilities.

Land-use data are collected on an annual basis in Metropolitan Toronto for spatial units termed 'basic planning units'. A basic planning unit corresponds almost exactly in spatial extent to a census tract. Hence, several census enumeration areas comprise a basic planning unit/census tract. This means that two different CEAs (the basic unit for sampling purposes) could conceivably have a different social status classification although the same land-use characteristics. In other words, the operational definition of a 'neighbourhood' for the land-use and neighbourhood social status measures refers to two different spatial units.

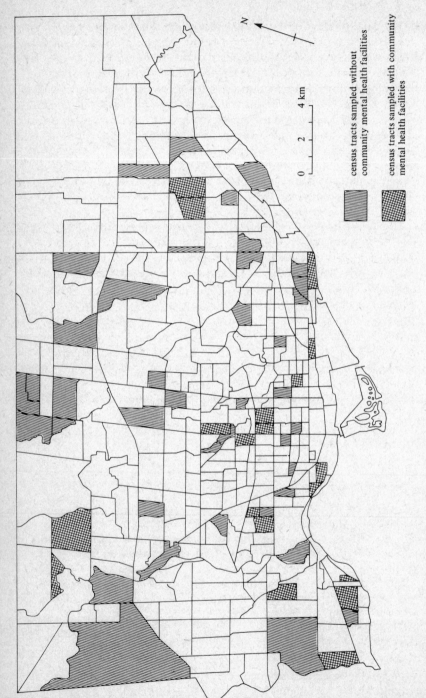

census tracts sampled without
community mental health facilities

census tracts sampled with community
mental health facilities

N

0   2   4 km

Figure 5.2. Sampled census tracts in Metropolitan Toronto.

This is a problem of data availability, since land-use information is not assembled in Metropolitan Toronto below the basic planning unit level. Faced with time and manpower restrictions, it was decided to use the available information (for 1978–1979) rather than survey each of the sixty-nine sampled enumeration areas for more precise land-use data. Absolute acreage figures were tabulated for seven different land uses for each basic planning unit and simple percentages were calculated for each category. The distribution of basic planning units/census tracts for which land-use information was collected is shown in figure 5.2, and the categories and their constituent land uses are given in table 5.7.

Neighbourhood social structure was measured in two ways. At the CEA level, social structure was defined in terms of the socioeconomic index used in the sample selection. At the census tract level, 1971 and 1976 census data were extracted for the fifty-eight tracts included in the combined with facilities and without facilities samples. Census tract measures were regarded as a better indicator of several area characteristics than measures defined at the CEA level since the CEA normally encompasses a very small geographic area. Census variables were selected to represent major demographic and social neighbourhood characteristics including age, education, mobility, ethnicity, marital status, homeownership and employment status. Comparison of the 1971 and 1976 data for variables collected in both years provided measures of growth and change for the sample neighbourhoods. The CEA socioeconomic index is used for the analysis of individual reactions to facilities (chapter 7); the census tract data are used in the analysis of community responses (chapter 10).

Table 5.7. Categories of land use.

Land use	Constituents
Residential	includes semidetached dwellings, multiple department dwellings, multiple other
Commercial	includes individual stores, shopping strips, shopping centres, car and other automotive sales, accommodation
Industrial	includes workshops, heavy industry, general industrial, other industrial storage buildings, storage yards
Institutional	includes places of worship, other assemblies, auditoriums, exhibits, schools, universities/colleges, hospitals, care/custody facilities, protection facilities, other facilities
Transportation and utilities	includes main buildings, open plants, depots, stations, parking, expressways, airports, hydro plants
Open space	includes parks, park reserves, golf courses, stadiums, cemeteries, other recreation facilities
Vacant	includes construction sites, vacant parcels of land, disused sites

5.4 Summary

In this chapter we have described the design of the Toronto study. The main data set required to test the theoretical model of individual response to neighbourhood mental health facilities was obtained by a questionnaire survey of Metropolitan Toronto residents conducted between June and October 1978. Two separate multistage cluster samples were drawn as the basis for data collection. The samples comprised areas with and without existing mental health facilities. The final sample totalled 1090 respondents, 702 from areas without facilities and 388 from areas with facilities. The questionnaire designed for the study contained a wide range of questions on general and specific reactions to the mentally ill and mental health facilities. Questions were included to provide information on each of the components of the model including beliefs, attitudes, behavioural intentions, and behaviour. The neighbourhood-level data needed for the study were obtained from land-use and census records. Information on housing transactions in areas with existing facilities and on matched control areas was collected from real estate records. These data are used to examine the effects of mental health facility locations on property values (see chapter 9).

Development of belief scales

Beliefs comprise a major component of our theoretical model and the analysis of nonuser response to mental health facilities required the development of new multiple item scales to measure two sets of salient beliefs: beliefs about the mentally ill, and neighbourhood beliefs. Although for our purposes these scales are a means to an end, in themselves they represent a significant methodological development, which it is important to describe before proceeding to the main analysis chapters. This chapter outlines scale construction and testing procedures. Scales for measuring beliefs about the mentally ill are described first, followed by scales for measuring neighbourhood beliefs.

6.1 Scales for measuring beliefs about the mentally ill
6.1.1 Scale selection
As discussed in chapter 4, previous research provides several different scaling instruments to measure beliefs about the mentally ill. We pointed out, however, that these scales are of questionable utility for a community-based study of beliefs held by the general public. There are two main reasons for questioning their use for our purposes. First, most were constructed prior to the widespread emergence of community-based mental health care and therefore do not tap the concepts and ideas associated with social psychiatry and community psychology. Second, most existing scales were constructed with professionals in mind as the potential respondents. As a result they tend to assume a psychiatric knowledge beyond what can be reasonably expected of a lay person. Our approach, therefore, has been to regard the best of the existing scales as a starting point for our own scale construction, recognizing the need for substantial revisions to deal with these two major concerns.

The 'opinions about mental illness' scales and the 'community mental health ideology' scale provided the most useful foundation for the development of our scales. The OMI, as probably the most widely used and best validated instrument, identifies important dimensions underlying personal beliefs about the mentally ill. The CMHI, given its focus on adherence to the general principle of community mental health, has perhaps the most direct relevance to our objectives. Given that our basic aim was to predict and explain public reactions to local mental health facilities, it was not judged necessary to construct scales to measure all possible belief dimensions, but rather to focus on those which are the most strongly evaluative and, hence, most likely to discriminate between those positively and those negatively disposed toward the mentally ill and mental health facilities. On this basis, two of the five OMI scales—mental hygiene ideology and interpersonal etiology—were dropped from consideration. These scales are also problematic because of the psychiatric knowledge they assume. The remaining three OMI scales—authoritarianism, benevolence, and social restrictiveness—and the CMHI scale were made the basis for our scale construction.

6.1.2 Scale construction

The initial item pool comprised forty Likert statements, ten for each of the four selected scales. Only seven of the forty statements came from the original OMI and CMHI scales: three for authoritarianism, two each for benevolence and social restrictiveness, and none for community mental health ideology. Four additional authoritarianism items came from the 'custodial mental illness' scale (CMI) developed by Gilbert and Levinson (1956). For the three OMI scales, the new statements do not alter significantly the content domains of the scales as originally conceived by Cohen and Struening (1964). Their effect is to emphasize those facets of the content domains which impinge most directly on community contact with the mentally ill. For the CMHI scale, the revisions are more fundamental because the original statements were clearly intended for application in a professional context, and, hence, a completely new set of statements was required for community-based research. These new statements shift the focus of the scale from the professional's adherence to the general principle of community mental health, as emphasized in the Baker and Schulberg scale, to the acceptance by the general population of mental health services and clients in the community. The themes expressed in the new scales are summarized in the following descriptions.

Sentiments embedded in the *authoritarianism* statements were: the need to hospitalize the mentally ill (for example, "As soon as a person shows signs of mental disturbance, he should be hospitalized"; the difference between the mentally ill and normal people (for example, "There is something about the mentally ill that makes it easy to tell them from normal people"); the importance of custodial care (for example, "Mental patients need the same kind of control and discipline as an untrained child"); and the cause of mental illness (for example, "The mentally ill are not to blame for their problems"). For *benevolence*, the sentiments were: the responsibility of society for the mentally ill (for example, "More tax money should be spent on the care and treatment of the mentally ill"); the need for sympathetic, kindly attitudes (for example, "The mentally ill have for too long been the subject of ridicule"); willingness to become personally involved (for example, "It is best to avoid anyone who has mental problems"); and anticustodial feelings (for example, "Our mental hospitals seem more like prisons than like places where the mentally ill can be cared for"). The *social restrictiveness* statements tapped the following themes: the dangerousness of the mentally ill (for example, "The mentally ill are a danger to themselves and those around them"); maintaining social distance (for example, "A woman would be foolish to marry a man who has suffered from mental illness, even though he seems fully recovered"); lack of responsibility (for example, "The mentally ill are very unpredictable and should not be given any responsibility"); and the normality of the mentally ill (for example, "Many people who have never had psychiatric treatment have more serious mental problems than many mental patients"). For the CMHI scale, statements expressed the following sentiments: the therapeutic value of the community (for example, "The best therapy for many mental patients is to be part of a normal community"); the impact of mental health facilities on residential neighbourhoods (for example, "Locating mental health facilities in a residential area downgrades the neighbourhood"); the danger to local residents posed by the mentally ill (for example, "It is frightening to think of people with mental problems living in residential neighbourhoods"); and acceptance of the principle of deinstitutionalized care (for example, "Mental hospitals have a very limited role to play in a civilized society").

6.1.3 Scale reliability and validity

Two separate tests were conducted to assess the reliability and validity of the statements and scales. The first was based on a group of first-year undergraduate students in urban geography ($N = 321$) at McMaster University, and the second on the respondents ($N = 54$) in a field pretest conducted by the York University Survey Research Centre. For both sets of data, item–total correlations and alpha coefficients [3] were calculated as measures of statement and scale reliability (Nunnally, 1967).

Table 6.1. Statement and scale reliabilities—the sizes of the data sets are: McMaster $N = 321$, York $N = 54$, final $N = 1090$. (Source: Taylor and Dear, 1981, page 229.)

Data set	Scale			
	authoritarianism	benevolence	social restrictiveness	community mental health ideology
Average item–scale R				
McMaster	0·27	0·46	0·38	0·45
York	0·29	0·27	0·40	0·25
Final	0·34	0·44	0·47	0·61
Range of item–scale Rs				
McMaster	0·15–0·44	0·31–0·35	0·15–0·57	−0·06–0·70
York	0·03–0·59	0·10–0·35	0·23–0·57	−0·06–0·64
Final	0·15–0·45	0·22–0·53	0·34–0·63	0·41–0·76
Alpha coefficient				
McMaster	0·58	0·79	0·70	0·77
York	0·62	0·58	0·59	0·53
Final	0·68	0·76	0·80	0·88

[3] The alpha coefficient is given by $\alpha = k\bar{r}_{ij}/[1 + (k-1)\bar{r}_{ij}]$, where k is the number of items, and $\bar{r}_{ij}$ is the average correlation between the items.

Table 6.2. Factor structure for the final scales used to measure beliefs about the mentally ill—factor loadings $>0 \cdot 40$ are underlined. The headings 1–4 refer to the relevant factors. (Source: Taylor and Dear, 1981, pages 230–231.)

Statement	1	2	3	4
Authoritarianism				
One of the main causes of mental illness is a lack of self-discipline and will power	0·51	0·02	−0·24	0·00
The best way to handle the mentally ill is to keep them behind locked doors	0·48	−0·18	−0·26	0·09
There is something about the mentally ill that makes it easy to tell them from normal people	0·52	−0·07	−0·09	0·12
As soon as a person shows signs of mental disturbance, he should be hospitalized	0·55	−0·06	0·05	0·24
Mental patients need the same kind of control and discipline as a young child	0·51	−0·13	−0·05	0·16
Mental illness is an illness like any other	0·08	−0·10	−0·22	0·18
The mentally ill should not be treated as outcasts of society	0·21	−0·25	−0·34	0·22
Less emphasis should be placed on protecting the public from the mentally ill	0·12	−0·19	−0·12	0·34
Mental hospitals are an outdated means of treating the mentally ill	0·03	−0·05	−0·01	0·47
Virtually anyone can become mentally ill	0·19	−0·11	−0·33	0·25
Benevolence				
The mentally ill have for too long been the subject of ridicule	−0·18	0·12	0·39	−0·35
More tax money should be spent on the care and treatment of the mentally ill	−0·00	0·21	0·54	−0·08
We need to adopt a far more tolerant attitude toward the mentally ill in our society	−0·13	0·21	0·51	−0·08
Our mental hospitals seem more like prisons than like places where the mentally ill can be cared for	−0·08	0·06	0·10	−0·43
We have a responsibility to provide the best possible care for the mentally ill	−0·07	0·12	0·60	−0·20
The mentally ill do not deserve our sympathy	−0·25	0·08	0·41	0·02
The mentally ill are a burden on society	−0·41	0·21	0·25	0·02
Increased spending on mental health services is a waste of tax dollars	−0·28	0·22	0·51	0·04
There are sufficient existing services for the mentally ill	−0·32	0·19	0·34	−0·13
It is best to avoid anyone who has mental problem problems	−0·57	0·21	0·34	−0·04
Social restrictiveness				
The mentally ill should not be given any responsibility	0·51	−0·14	−0·23	0·16
The mentally ill should be isolated from the rest of the community	0·55	−0·32	−0·23	0·16

Table 6.2 (continued)

Statement	1	2	3	4
Social restrictiveness (continued)				
A woman would be foolish to marry a man who has suffered from mental illness, even though he seems fully recovered	0·52	−0·24	−0·11	0·06
I would not want to live next door to someone who has been mentally ill	0·54	−0·46	−0·16	0·15
Anyone with a history of mental problems should be excluded from taking public office	0·48	−0·20	−0·12	0·17
The mentally ill should not be denied their individual rights	0·23	−0·15	−0·22	0·26
Mental patients should be encouraged to assume the responsibilities of normal life	0·12	−0·13	−0·34	0·30
No one has the right to exclude the mentally ill from their neighbourhood	0·15	−0·39	−0·23	0·20
The mentally ill are far less of a danger than most people suppose	0·26	−0·22	−0·14	0·44
Most women who were once patients in a mental hospital can be trusted as baby sitters	0·34	−0·20	−0·04	0·28
Community mental health ideology				
Residents should accept the location of mental health facilities in their neighbourhood to serve the needs of the local community	−0·09	0·65	0·29	−0·16
The best therapy for many mental patients is to be part of a normal community	−0·21	0·37	0·23	−0·30
As far as possible mental health services should be provided through community-based facilities	−0·06	0·33	0·20	−0·35
Locating mental health services in residential neighbourhoods does not endanger local residents	−0·21	0·58	0·16	−0·29
Residents have nothing to fear from people coming into their neighbourhood to obtain mental health services	−0·20	0·55	0·17	−0·23
Mental health facilities should be kept out of residential neighbourhoods	−0·38	0·67	0·22	−0·10
Local residents have good reason to resist the location of mental health services in their neighbourhood	−0·39	0·59	0·21	−0·14
Having mental patients living within residential neighbourhoods might be good therapy, but the risks to residents are too great	−0·52	0·45	0·12	−0·15
It is frightening to think of people with mental problems living in residential neighbourhoods	−0·56	0·44	0·15	−0·12
Locating mental health facilities in a residential area downgrades the neighbourhood	−0·37	0·56	0·22	−0·06
Variance accounted for by each factor (%)	28·1	5·5	4·2	3·9

If we consider the results from both samples (table 6.1), the alpha coefficients are for all four scales above 0·50, which can be regarded as a satisfactory (though modest) level of reliability in the early stages of scale construction. The coefficients are notably higher for the McMaster student group for three of the scales (except authoritarianism) which have relatively strong values of alpha above 0·70. Although the scales are in general satisfactory, inspection of the statement–scale correlations showed a number of statements which made very little contribution to their parent scale. These statements were replaced by statements expressing similar sentiments to those contained in statements more strongly correlated with total scale scores. In addition, two statements on the social restrictiveness scale were replaced to eliminate unecessary repetition. It is important to note that all of the statements included in the item pool from the original OMI scales were strongly correlated with total scale scores and hence were retained in the final scales. This finding is confirmation that our revised versions of the three OMI scales have the same content domains as the original scales.

The same statistics were calculated to test the reliability and validity of the revised scales by use of the full Toronto data set ($N = 1090$). The alpha coefficients (table 6.1) are, in all cases but one, higher than the pretest values, the one exception being on the benevolence scale where the coefficient for the final scale is marginally lower than for the McMaster pretest. Three of the four scales have high reliability: CMHI ($\alpha = 0·88$), social restrictiveness ($\alpha = 0·80$), and benevolence ($\alpha = 0·76$). The coefficient for authoritarianism ($\alpha = 0·68$), though lower, is still satisfactory. These increases in the alpha values reflect the general strengthening of the item–total correlation for statements retained from the pretest, and the improvement due to the replacement of the statements shown to be weak in the pretest results.

The construct validity of the final scales was assessed by testing their empirical reproducibility by means of factor analysis. A four-factor orthogonal solution accounting for 42% of the variance was obtained (table 6.2). Factor scores were calculated and correlated with the raw scores on the four a priori scales. The matrix of correlations among the a priori and factor scales (table 6.3) is revealing in two respects. First, it shows a high degree of intercorrelation among the a priori scales. The lowest correlation is −0·63 between authoritarianism and benevolence, and the highest is −0·77 between social restrictiveness and CMHI. These coefficients can, in part, be compared with those reported in previous studies using the OMI (Fracchia et al, 1972). In general, the correlations in this case are higher, possibly reflecting the fact that the distinctions between the scales are not as clear to the general population as they are to the professionals who were respondents in the earlier studies. More importantly, the difference may also reflect the revisions made to the scales for this study.

Second, the correlation matrix (table 6.3) shows a reasonable degree of correspondence between the a priori and factor scales, which is the desired result from a construct validity standpoint. The CMHI scale is strongly identified with the second factor ($r = 0 \cdot 86$), and the benevolence scale almost as strongly with the third factor ($r = 0 \cdot 81$). Authoritarianism and social restrictiveness are approximately equally correlated with the first factor and to a lesser extent with the fourth factor. This provides some evidence that these two scales perhaps represent a single dimension. They are, however, treated separately in the subsequent analyses. The remaining coefficients in the lower right of the matrix show the low correlation among the factor scales. This is an artifact of the algorithm which forces independence between the factors within an orthogonal solution.

Table 6.3. Scale validities[a] (Pearson correlation coefficients) for the final data set— $N = 1090$. (Source: Taylor and Dear, 1981, page 232.)

	A	B	SR	CMHI	F1	F2	F3	F4
Authoritarianism	–	−0·63	0·72	−0·64	0·73	−0·25	−0·34	0·51
Benevolence		–	−0·65	0·65	−0·45	0·33	0·81	−0·31
Social restrictiveness			–	−0·77	0·72	−0·49	−0·32	0·46
Community health health ideology				–	−0·49	0·86	0·33	−0·34
Factor 1					–	−0·13	−0·07	0·06
Factor 2						–	0·10	−0·11
Factor 3							–	−0·12
Factor 4								–

[a] The column headings are abbreviations of the row headings.

6.1.4 Summary

The development of new scales to measure community beliefs about the mentally ill originated in the geographic problem of explaining spatial variations in public response to mental health facilities. Four existing scales were the basis for constructing a new set of scales representing four dimensions of community beliefs: authoritarianism, benevolence, social restrictiveness, and community mental health ideology. These scales differ from the originals in two main respects: first, by their emphasis on those facets of the content domain of each scale which relate most directly to community contact with the mentally ill; and, second, by the statements being worded with a general public rather than professional sample in mind.

The internal and external validity of the new scales was extensively analysed by use of the pretest and final data sets for the Toronto study. Weak items identified in the pretest were replaced prior to the major data-collection phase. High levels of internal validity were shown for the final scales based on item–scale correlations, alpha coefficients, and factor analysis. External validity was examined in two ways within the theoretical framework for the Toronto study (see chapter 7). Construct validity was assessed by analysing relationships between the belief scales and a range of personal characteristics. Predictive validity was tested by analysing relationships between the scales and various measures of response to mental health facilities. In both cases, the strength, direction, and consistency of the relationships provides strong support for the external validity of the new scales.

The new scales meet the immediate need for reliable and valid measures of beliefs about the mentally ill for use in the Toronto study. From a longer-term perspective, we hope that these scales go some way toward meeting the need for sound measures of public beliefs about the mentally ill created by the shift to community-based mental health care. We hope that future applications of these scales beyond the Toronto study will further strengthen their validity.

6.2 Scales for measuring neighbourhood beliefs

In chapter 2 we argued that neighbourhood beliefs influence attitudes to facilities because, together with beliefs about facilities, they determine an individual's perception of the suitability of the neighbourhood as a facility location. The questionnaire provides measures of neighbourhood and facility beliefs which use the same seventy-eight-item adjective check list. For analysis purposes, these data were reduced to a set of six scale scores representing different dimensions of respondents' beliefs about the suitability of their neighbourhood as a location for a facility. This section outlines the development of these six scales.

6.2.1 Scale selection

The items for the neighbourhood and facility check list were selected to represent six underlying a priori scales: activity, evaluation, safety, integration, design, and predictability (table 6.4). An approximately equal number of negative and positive adjectives were selected for each scale. The choice of scales was based on past research in environmental perception in general, and in public facility perception in particular. *Activity* and *evaluation* are generally recognized as two important dimensions on which perceptions are structured (Osgood et al, 1957). Thouez (1975) suggested that a third dimension, *predictability* (familiarity) was important in forming perceptions of public facilities. The *safety, integration*, and *design* scales were also included for their judged relevance to perceptions of mental health facilities. The dimensions of *integration* and *design* are important concerns about the facility itself, and the dimensions of *safety* and *predictability* are important concerns about the mentally ill.

The items were initially culled from Craik's 300-item *Environmental Adjective Check List* (Craik, 1971). Many of Craik's adjectives were rejected either on the basis of being inappropriate for the stimuli of interest, or because of being too uncommon in everyday usage to be included in a general population survey. A number of adjectives not in Craik's list were added as being particularly appropriate. In short, a rational, intuitive approach formed the basis for item selection for each of the six scales.

Table 6.4. A priori adjective scales. (Source: Isaak et al, 1980, page 239.)

Activity	Evaluation	Safety	Integration	Design	Predictability
calm	appealing	friendly	harmonious	organized	familiar
peaceful	attractive	human	inconspicuous	planned	normal
quiet	cheerful	inviting	unnoticeable	private	ordinary
relaxed	clean	orderly	hidden	residential	permanent
deserted	good	safe	small	accessible	predictable
slow	interesting	sociable		convenient	stable
		sympathetic		well-	
		welcoming	conspicuous	maintained	
active	bad		inconsistent		odd
busy	depressing		contrasting	chaotic	strange
congested	dirty	dangerous	institutional	confusing	uncertain
noisy	repellant	disturbing	out-of-place	commercial	unfamiliar
crowded	rundown	frightening	noticeable	public	unnatural
fast	ugly	inhuman	visible	unplanned	unusual
	unpleasant	tense	big		
		threatening			
		unfriendly			
		insecure			

6.2.2 Scale validation

The internal validity of the a priori scales, was assessed by a factor analysis of the mental health facility check list data from the final Toronto study sample ($N = 1090$). Each adjective was scored 0 if not checked and 1 if checked. Each, therefore, represents a dummy interval variable legitimate for input to a parametric procedure such as factor analysis.

A six-factor orthogonal solution was obtained, accounting for $36 \cdot 3\%$ of the variance. The six factor scales are listed in table 6.5. The first two scales represent general perceptions or evaluations of mental health facilities. These scales are broad in scope in that they comprise adjectives pertaining to the safety associated with facility users, and to the design and integration of the facility itself. The fact that the first scale combines positive adjectives and the second combines negative ones suggests that there is a basic dichotomous structure to general evaluations of mental health facilities. The third scale is a design scale representing perceptions of mental health facilities that fit an institutional stereotype. The fourth

Table 6.5. Factor scales (adjectives with factor loadings between ±0·200 were not included).

Adjective	Factor loading	Adjective	Factor loading	Adjective	Factor loading
Factor 1: Positive evaluation					
friendly	0·717	appealing	0·606	accessible	0·495
cheerful	0·709	good	0·599	residential	0·481
welcoming	0·696	convenient	0·594	permanent	0·439
relaxed	0·688	clean	0·585	sympathetic	0·359
inviting	0·679	normal	0·549	ordinary	0·355
sociable	0·660	orderly	0·547	visible	0·345
harmonious	0·657	organized	0·530	public	0·325
interesting	0·643	planned	0·527	predictable	0·305
well-maintained	0·634	human	0·525	institutional	−0·264
stable	0·622	quiet	0·511	disturbing	−0·207
attractive	0·618	familiar	0·508	depressing	−0·326
safe	0·608	calm	0·497		
peaceful	0·607	active	0·497		
Factor 2: Negative evaluation					
bad	0·614	depressing	0·418	strange	0·346
dirty	0·591	confusing	0·413	congested	0·338
ugly	0·575	unnatural	0·411	tense	0·305
dangerous	0·528	threatening	0·411	odd	0·282
unpleasant	0·502	unfriendly	0·400	crowded	0·281
frightening	0·490	insecure	0·399	unplanned	0·219
repellent	0·481	out-of-place	0·397	uncertain	0·238
disturbing	0·453	chaotic	0·356	conspicuous	0·236
inhuman	0·433	noisy	0·353	inconsistent	0·217
rundown	0·419	deserted	0·348		
Factor 3: Design					
busy	0·578	confusing	0·338	hidden	0·221
crowded	0·565	tense	0·336	active	0·219
congested	0·453	noisy	0·275	public	0·215
institutional	0·407	inconsistent	0·249	fast	0·191
depressing	0·368	big	0·240	calm	−0·222
chaotic	0·338	commercial	0·222		
Factor 4: Safety					
strange	0·542	tense	0·295	slow	0·220
unusual	0·464	unnatural	0·258	out-of-place	0·212
odd	0·426	confusing	0·249	frightening	0·211
unfamiliar	0·344	threatening	0·247	inhuman	0·210
insecure	0·338	disturbing	0·227	institutional	0·201
Factor 5: Positive integration					
inconspicuous	0·358	ordinary	0·271	residential	0·230
private	0·355	predictable	0·270	stable	0·209
quiet	0·337	unnoticeable	0·268	small	0·207
hidden	0·333	inconsistent	0·237		
Factor 6: Negative integration					
noticeable	0·403	conspicuous	0·316	institutional	0·212
permanent	0·383	predictable	0·281	contrasting	0·212
visible	0·382	disturbing	0·259		

scale is a safety scale representing perceptions of the mentally ill. The fifth and sixth scales are integration scales representing perceptions of how well mental health facilities are integrated into residential neighbourhoods. Again, the fact that the fifth and sixth combine positive and negative objectives, respectively, suggests a basic dichotomy in perceptions of mental health facilities measured on the dimension of integration.

The factor scales are somewhat different from the a priori scales. Interscale correlations were calculated, based on standardized scores on each scale, and are summarized in table 6.6. The a priori safety, evaluation, design, and predictability scales correlate with the first factor scale, positive evaluation (safety 0·84, evaluation 0·80, design 0·72, and predictability 0·62). The same a priori scales correlate on the second factor scale, negative evaluation. These correlations are negative and weaker (safety −0·79, evaluation −0·77, design −0·65, predictability −0·57).

Although none of the a priori scales correlate highly on the third factor scale, negative design, correlations are highest for the a priori activity (−0·68) and design (−0·59) scales. The a priori safety scale has the highest correlation on the negative safety scale (−0·78). None of the a priori scales correlate highly with the fifth factor scale, positive integration. The highest correlation is for the a priori integration scale (0·32). Finally, the sixth factor scale, negative integration, is highly correlated with only the a priori integration scale (−0·73).

Overall, the six a priori scales have been compressed into four broader factor scales, or dimensions. The first two factor scales, general evaluations, comprise many more adjectives than the a priori evaluation scale. This suggests that general evaluations of mental health facilities are based on many different considerations, including safety, integration and design. The design factor scale is a combination of the a priori design and activity scales. The factor and a priori safety scales correspond, as do the factor

Table 6.6. A priori and factor scale correlations[a].

A priori scales	Empirical scales					
	positive evaluation	negative evaluation	negative design	negative safety	positive integration	negative integration
Activity	0·3970	−0·4321	−0·6831	−0·2939	0·2204	0·2431
Evaluation	0·8045	−0·7725	−0·5749	−0·6466	ns	−0·3774
Safety	0·8379	−0·7932	−0·5640	−0·7774	0·0630[***]	−0·4476
Integration	0·4506	−0·4621	−0·4904	−0·5121	0·3157	−0·7332
Design	0·7204	−0·6476	−0·5884	−0·5744	0·2158	−0·2914
Predictability	0·6194	−0·5668	−0·3544	−0·6516	0·2749	−0·1374

[a] ns denotes not significant, [***] denotes significant at the 0·05 level, and all other correlations are significant at the 0·001 level.

and a priori integration scales. Although the factor-analysis results only
partially validate the a priori scales, they were retained in subsequent
analysis for two reasons. First, they have greater face validity and
intelligibility than the factor scales. Second, the factor structure may have
been distorted by the relatively large number of adjectives which were very
infrequently checked and hence had very skewed frequency distributions.

6.2.3 Standardization of scale scores

For analytical purposes, standardized scores were calculated on the six
scales to take account of variations in the total number of adjectives
checked. The standardization procedure follows that adopted by Gough
and Heilbrun (1965). The first step was to calculate the raw score for
each individual on each scale both for the facility and for the neighbourhood check lists. The raw scale score was equal to the number of positive
adjectives minus the number of negative adjectives checked. The raw
scores were then standardized according to the following formula:

$$\text{standard score} = \frac{\text{raw score} - \text{mean raw score}}{\text{standard deviation of mean raw score}} \times 10 + 50 \, .$$

To calculate the standard scores, the population was divided into four
percentile groups of equal size for both checklists, based on the total
number of adjectives checked. The mean and standard deviation of the
group raw scores were then used in the formula, rather than the mean and
standard deviation for the total population. Gough and Heilbrun further
split the population according to sex and calculated separate scores for
each. As a t-test revealed no significant difference in the number of
adjectives checked by male and female respondents in these data, this
distinction was not made.

These calculations resulted in each individual having a standard score on
each scale both for the facility and for the neighbourhood. The standard
scores all ranged from 0 to 100 with a mean standard score on each scale
of 50. The actual score number represents the degree of 'positiveness' or
'negativeness' of the perceptions of the individual on a particular scale.
For example, an individual with a standard score of 62 on the evaluation
scale for the neighbourhood can be said to have a higher than average
neighbourhood evaluation. If the individual had a score of 35 on the
safety scale for the facility, it could be said that the individual had a
lower than average perception of the safety of mental health facilities and
their users.

One further step was involved to obtain appropriate neighbourhood
belief measures for use in the main analysis. Recall that we previously
stated that we required measures of the respondents' beliefs about the
suitability of the neighbourhood as a location for a facility. A simple but
reasonable method to obtain these measures is to calculate the difference

between the standardized scores on each scale for the neighbourhood and the facility. By subtracting the neighbourhood score from the facility score on each scale, six measures of beliefs about the suitability of the neighbourhood as a facility location were obtained for each respondent. A positive scale score therefore indicated that an individual held a more positive perception of a mental health facility than the neighbourhood and a negative score the reverse. Positive scale scores characterize respondents who believe their neighbourhood to be a suitable location for a facility and negative scores represent those who believe it to be unsuitable.

6.3 Summary

The important role played by beliefs as the antecedents of attitudes and behaviour in our theoretical model emphasizes the need for reliable and valid instruments to measure them. A new set of scales was developed to measure beliefs about mental illness and the mentally ill. Although initially based on three of Cohen and Struening's OMI scales and the Baker and Schulberg CMHI scale, the new scales represent wholesale revisions of the originals with the aims of focussing on community-based mental health care and of designing statements suited to the general public rather than professional respondents. Results from the reliability and validity tests were encouraging and suggest that future applications of the scales are warranted.

The development of scales to measure beliefs about the suitability of the neighbourhood as a facility location required a novel approach given that no precedent exists in the literature. Accepting that these beliefs derive from the integration of general neighbourhood perceptions and mental health facility perceptions, the approach adopted involved measuring both sets of perceptions by use of the same adjective check list. Responses were reduced to standardized scores on six scales which had been partially validated by the results of factor analysis. The required belief measures were then calculated as the difference between the standardized scale scores for the neighbourhood and the facility. We recognize that these scales are experimental and may need considerable refinement in the course of future investigations. Nevertheless, they provide a systematically and logically derived instrument for measuring important though quite intangible beliefs.

7 Individual response to neighbourhood mental health facilities

The major objective of the Toronto study was to investigate the factors affecting public reaction to neighbourhood mental health facilities. The framework for that investigation is contained in the theoretical model presented in chapter 2. In this chapter the main relationships in the model are analyzed. As previously described, the model has six major components: external variables, beliefs, attitudes, behavioural intentions, behaviour, and outcomes. The Toronto data allow us to test the relationships among the first four. Too few survey respondents had actually taken any actions in response to mental health facilities to make it feasible to include behavioural measures in the analytical design. The results are discussed in three sections: the relationships between external variables and beliefs, the relationships between beliefs and attitudes, and the relationships between attitudes and behavioural intentions.

7.1 External variables and beliefs
In the model, three sets of external variables are linked to the formation of salient beliefs. These are facility characteristics, personal characteristics, and neighbourhood characteristics. These sets of factors play an external role in the sense that they are outside the psychological process leading from belief formation to behaviour. Yet their inclusion in the analysis is very important because they potentially increase the explanatory power of the model by indicating the antecedents of beliefs. Three groups of relationships are examined in this section. We first consider the effects of facility characteristics on beliefs about facility impacts. The relationships between personal characteristics and beliefs about facility impacts are then examined. Finally, the links between personal characteristics and beliefs about the mentally ill are considered. We do not deal here with the effects of external variables on beliefs about the neighbourhood. Neighbourhood beliefs are included in the later analysis of the link between beliefs and attitudes.

7.1.1 Facility characteristics and beliefs about facility impacts
The Toronto survey sample was designed to include respondents living in areas in which different types of mental health facility already exist. The hope was that this design would allow us to examine the effects of facility characteristics on beliefs about facility impacts. However, the data showed a fundamental problem. An unexpectedly small number of respondents in the with facilities sample were aware of the existence of a mental health facility in their neighbourhood. Of the 388 respondents selected because they had a facility within approximately 400 metres of their home, only 83 indicated awareness of the existence of a facility in their neighbour-

hood. Closer inspection of the data showed that in fact only 33 of the 83 were aware of the facility closest to their home which was the basis for their inclusion in the sample. The obvious question is why there is such a low level of awareness. The most likely explanation has to do with the invisibility of many of the facilities. In the case of the residential care facilities, the group homes or commercial boarding homes are typically indistinguishable from neighbouring housing and, therefore, unless specific incidents have occurred to attract public attention, it is very likely that their existence could remain unknown except to those living very close by. Equally, many of the nonresidential facilities are inconspicuous. Social-therapeutic centres, for example, are commonly incorporated within existing facilities such as churches and community centres and, again, easily go unnoticed. The only high-profile facilities are drop-in centres using store-front operations, but these are very few in number in Toronto and are usually located in commercial areas where their presence could easily be overlooked.

This very low level of facility awareness severely limits any assessment of the effects of facility characteristics on beliefs about impacts. We necessarily had to revise our analytical approach accordingly and decided simply to examine whether facility awareness regardless of facility type affected beliefs. For this analysis the aware group was defined as all respondents who indicated awareness of a facility in their neighbourhood irrespective of the facility they named and regardless of whether they were nominally in the with facilities sample or not. On this basis, there were 139 respondents aware of a facility and 951 unaware.

Beliefs about facility impacts were measured in terms of the respondent's ratings on twelve semantic differential scales. For those unaware of the facility, the ratings represent beliefs about the impacts a mental health facility *would have* on the neighbourhood, and for those aware, they represent beliefs about the impacts a facility *has had*. The data are treated in two ways. For descriptive purposes, the seven-point rating scale is reduced to three categories: negative, neutral, and positive beliefs about impacts. To test for significant differences in median ratings between the aware and unaware groups, the full scale information is used.

The percentage distributions for the negative, neutral, and positive categories show that for both groups and for all twelve impact scales the modal response is neutral (table 7.1). Further, with the exception of beliefs about neighbourhood image and neighbourhood quantity, the percentage neutral is higher for the aware group suggesting that experience of a facility may lead to less extreme beliefs. In general, the percentage expressing negative beliefs is lower for the aware group; again the exception is for neighbourhood image, which together with the previous findings implies that experience tends to neutralize negative expectations. The differences between the two groups in the percentages expressing positive beliefs about impacts is consistently small. Experience has not, therefore, generated any sizeable increase in positive feelings about facilites. The expectation that mental health facilities are generally unwanted by local residents finds support in the fact that the percentage negative exceeds the percentage positive in all but two cases. These both occur for the aware group, where for residential character and property taxes more respondents expressed positive than negative beliefs. Insofar, therefore, that awareness of facilities has any effect on beliefs about facility impacts, it is in the direction of softening rather than hardening residents' views. However, we cannot infer a cause and effect relationship between awareness and facility perceptions because awareness covaries with other potentially salient variables, for example, residential location.

The statistical tests revealed significant differences between median ratings for the two groups for two of the twelve scales: traffic volumes and property taxes. The direction of the differences again shows more positive beliefs for the aware group. Although these differences are significant in statistical terms, they are small and we are led to the overall conclusion that the presence of a facility has no strong effect on people's beliefs about impacts. To the extent that the data show any trend, they suggest that the anticipated impacts are worse than those actually experienced.

Table 7.1. Anticipated externality impact of a potential mental health facility—expressed as percentages. (Source: Dear et al, 1980, page 347.)

Impact variable	Anticipated effect					
	negative		neutral		positive	
	unaware	aware	unaware	aware	unaware	aware
Property value	46	42	45	54	8	4
Traffic volumes[a]	43	19	52	76	4	5
Resident satisfaction	39	35	39	49	22	16
Resident propensity to migrate	37	28	46	54	18	18
Neighbourhood image	32	32	48	45	20	23
Noise levels	31	22	58	65	12	13
Neighbourhood quality	28	25	52	52	20	22
Residential character	29	23	48	53	24	25
Attraction of undesirable nonresidents	27	23	61	69	12	9
Personal safety	25	21	60	65	15	15
Property taxes[b]	23	13	64	72	13	15
Visual appearance	20	19	63	66	17	15

[a] Difference between aware and unaware groups significant at less than the 0·01 level.
[b] Difference between aware and unaware groups significant at less than the 0·05 level.

7.1.2 Personal characteristics and beliefs about facility impacts

The questionnaire survey yielded a wide range of information on the personal characteristics of respondents. Preliminary analysis served to reduce the number of variables to a small subset which showed the strongest relationships with beliefs. Five variables were included in the analysis of the effects of personal characteristics on facility impacts: age, education level, tenure status, church attendance, and familiarity with the mentally ill. These five represent the major dimensions of demographic and social variation among respondents. For this analysis the impact scales were combined to produce an overall measure of the respondent's beliefs about facilities. The reliability of the composite scale was assessed by means of the standard measures of item–total correlations and alpha coefficient. The highest value of alpha (0·86) was obtained when composite scores were calculated over eleven scales, omitting the property tax scale which showed a low item–total correlation.

The relationships between the five personal characteristics and the composite belief scale were tested in a correlation analysis with tenure status, church attendance, and familiarity with the mentally ill being included as dummy variables. The results (table 7.2) show significant relationships for three of the five variables: age, tenure status, and familiarity with the mentally ill. In each case the relationship was in the hypothesized direction. The negative correlation on age shows that older respondents generally perceived facilities as having a more negative impact. For tenure status, the negative correlation indicates that owners have more negative beliefs than renters. The positive relationship with familiarity with mental illness shows as expected that those who had direct experience of mental illness among their family or friends hold more positive beliefs than those without such experience.

The overall conclusion from this part of the analysis is that the link between personal characteristics and beliefs about facility impacts is confirmed. At the same time we recognize that the significant relationships based on the correlation coefficients are quite weak and are limited to only three indicators.

Table 7.2. Personal characteristics and beliefs about facility impacts (figures are Pearson correlation coefficients).

Personal characteristics	Composite belief scale
Age	−0·17*
Education level	0·01
Tenure status	−0·17*
Church attendance	−0·05
Familiarity with mental illness	0·13*

* Significant beyond the 0·001 level.

7.1.3 Personal characteristics and beliefs about the mentally ill

The relationships between personal characteristics and beliefs about the mentally ill was the focus of more detailed analysis because previous research (see chapter 4) suggests that these beliefs are influenced by a combination of several variables. Two analytical approaches were adopted. The first tests the relationships between beliefs and each personal characteristic separately. The second involves a regression analysis to assess the degree to which beliefs about the mentally ill can be predicted by a linear combination of population characteristics.

The effects of fourteen different variables on beliefs about the mentally ill were examined. Demographic characteristics were measured by four variables: sex, age, marital status, and number of children in three age groups (under 6, 6 to 18, and over 18). Socioeconomic status was measured in conventional terms by education level, occupational status (both respondent and head of household), and household income, and, in addition, by tenure status. Personality variables were not measured directly. A proxy measure was included in terms of church attendance and denominational affiliation. Also included was a measure of familiarity with mental illness based on whether the respondent or his/her friends or relatives had ever used mental health services of any kind. Beliefs about the mentally ill were measured on the four scales described in detail in chapter 6, namely: authoritarianism, benevolence, social restrictiveness, and community mental health ideology.

The variables used in the analysis represent different levels of measurement: nominal, ordinal, and interval/ratio. The specific measurement properties of the paired combination of variables determines the statistical test used. The belief scales are assumed to have interval properties. Tests which relate beliefs to population characteristics with nominal properties are based on a difference of means test (t-test) where the characteristic has two categories (for example, sex), and a one-way analysis of variance (F-test) where there are more than two categories (for example, marital status). Relationships between population characteristics measured on an ordinal scale (for example, household income) and beliefs about the mentally ill are tested by nonparametric correlation (Kendall's tau). Finally, relationships involving characteristics with interval properties (for example, age) are tested by parametric correlation (Pearson's r).

Five of the six demographic variables examined show relatively strong relationships with the four belief scales, the exception being number of children over eighteen years of age (table 7.3). Consistent with previous studies, older residents report less sympathetic beliefs about the mentally ill. This pattern occurs for all four scales. Older respondents in the Toronto sample are, in general, more authoritarian, less benevolent, more socially restrictive and less community mental health oriented in their views.

Stronger effects for sex are found for these data than those reported in previous studies. The direction of the effect shows more sympathetic beliefs among female respondents. This emerges on three of the four scales. No significant difference occurs on social restrictiveness.

Highly significant differences are found among marital status groups on all four scales. Examination of the group means on each scale reveals the pattern of the effect. A basic distinction emerges between the married and widowed groups and those single, separated, or divorced, the former expressing the less sympathetic beliefs on each of the four scales. These differences in part reflect the age variation already observed and the effects of number and ages of children.

The number of children under six years of age and between six and eighteen years of age show very similar effects, the latter being marginally stronger. In both cases, respondents with children in these age groups are generally more authoritarian and socially restrictive and correspondingly less benevolent and community mental health oriented. The lack of significant effects for number of children over eighteen years of age supports the expectation that parents with older families will have fewer concerns about the mentally ill and their children's possible contact with them.

Taken together, these results indicate that the effects of demographic characteristics on beliefs about the mentally ill are both statistically significant and consistent in their direction. The variables included here, excepting sex, represent in combination a measure of life-cycle status. The combined effects of these variables is tested within the regression analysis reported later in the section (see table 7.6).

Table 7.3. Effects of demographic variables on beliefs about the mentally ill. (Source: Taylor and Dear, 1981, page 233.)

Demographic variables	Belief scales			
	authoritarianism	benevolence	social restrictiveness	CMHI
Age [a]	$0 \cdot 20^{*}$	$-0 \cdot 18^{*}$	$0 \cdot 32^{*}$	$-0 \cdot 21^{*}$
Sex [b]	$2 \cdot 65^{**}$	$-4 \cdot 56^{*}$	$1 \cdot 82^{ns}$	$-3 \cdot 02^{**}$
Marital status [c]	$10 \cdot 87^{*}$	$6 \cdot 12^{*}$	$16 \cdot 42^{*}$	$12 \cdot 13^{*}$
Children (<6) [a,d]	$0 \cdot 08^{**}$	$-0 \cdot 09^{**}$	$0 \cdot 07^{**}$	$-0 \cdot 11^{*}$
Children (6–18) [a,d]	$0 \cdot 08^{**}$	$-0 \cdot 09^{**}$	$0 \cdot 10^{*}$	$-0 \cdot 13^{*}$
Children (>18) [a,d]	$0 \cdot 06^{***}$	$-0 \cdot 03^{ns}$	$0 \cdot 03^{ns}$	$-0 \cdot 04^{ns}$

[a] Tested by Pearson's r.   [b] Tested by t-statistic.
[c] Tested by F-statistic.   [d] Number of children in age group.
[*] Significant at the $0 \cdot 001$ level.   [**] Significant at the $0 \cdot 01$ level.
[***] Significant at the $0 \cdot 05$ level.   [ns] Not significant at the $0 \cdot 05$ level.

Four of the five socioeconomic measures show strong and consistent relationships with the belief scales, the exception being household income (table 7.4). The observed direction of the relationships confirms previous findings in that more sympathetic beliefs are characteristic of higher status residents. This conclusion applies where status is measured either in educational or in occupational terms, although it is noted that the relationships are somewhat stronger for the education variable. Relationships with income, the third conventional measure of socioeconomic status, are weaker and for two scales, benevolence and CMHI, are not significant. This finding indicates that household income varies somewhat differently within the population than do education or occupation and that income is the least effective as a discriminator of beliefs about the mentally ill.

The significant effect of tenure status confirms the expectation that owners generally hold less sympathetic beliefs than renters, which possibly reflects their greater vested interest to protect their daily-life environment. Tenure effects are, however, more reliably assessed when controlling for other factors (for example, life-cycle stage) with which tenure typically covaries. The subsequent regression analysis provides a controlled test.

Church attendance and familiarity with mental health care show significant relationships with all four belief scales (table 7.5). Religious denomination has a significant effect on only the authoritarianism and benevolence scales. The direction of the effect for church attendance is that regular attenders are on average less sympathetic in their views, tending to be more authoritarian and socially restrictive and less benevolent and community mental health oriented. As could be expected, regular attenders, in general, hold more conservative views. Among attenders there are, however, significant denominational differences for two of the scales.

Table 7.4. Effects of socioeconomic variables on beliefs about the mentally ill. (Source: Taylor and Dear, 1981, page 234.)

Socioeconomic variables	Belief scales			
	authoritarianism	benevolence	social restrictiveness	CMHI
Education[a]	-0.27^*	0.17^*	-0.22^*	0.16^*
Occupation (respondent)[a]	-0.21^*	0.09^*	-0.12^*	0.08^*
Occupation (head)[a]	-0.19^*	0.08^*	-0.10^*	0.08^*
Household income[a]	0.11^*	0.03^{ns}	-0.06^{**}	0.01^{ns}
Tenure[b]	-3.64^*	4.60^*	-5.25^*	7.35^*

[a] Tested by Kendall's tau. [b] Tested by t-statistic.
* Significant at the 0.001 level. ** Significant at the 0.01 level.
^{ns} Not significant at the 0.05 level.

Of the thirteen major denominational groups distinguished in the coding of the data, the Pentecostal and Greek Orthodox groups emerge as the most authoritarian in contrast to the Baptists and Salvation Army who expressed the least authoritarian views. Correspondingly, the Baptists, together with the United Church adherents, held the most benevolent beliefs, again in contrast to the least benevolent views of the Pentecostal and Greek Orthodox members.

In terms of familiarity with mental health care, respondents who themselves had used mental health services or whose friends or relatives had used them expressed more sympathetic beliefs on all four scales. Personal experience of mental health care, whether direct or indirect, therefore has a significant effect on subsequent beliefs about the mentally ill and the provision of mental health services.

The second stage of the analysis involved calculating multiple regression equations to predict scores on the four belief scales. The independent variables were selected on the basis of two criteria: first, to maximize explanatory power by including variables shown by the previous analysis to be most strongly related to beliefs; second, to minimize collinearity by excluding variables highly correlated with variables already selected for inclusion. On these grounds the set of independent variables was restricted to three demographic characteristics—age, sex, and number of children six to eighteen years of age; two socioeconomic measures—education level and tenure status; and two belief measures—church attendance and familiarity with mental health care. Four of the seven variables (sex, tenure status, church attendance, and familiarity with mental health care) have only nominal measurement properties and are therefore included as dummy variables in the regression analysis.

A stepwise regression was performed such that at each step the independent variable accounting for the maximum residual variation in the

Table 7.5. Effects of other variables on beliefs about the mentally ill. (Source: Taylor and Dear, 1981, page 235.)

Variables	Belief scales			
	authoritarianism	benevolence	social restrictiveness	CMHI
Church attendance[a]	6·07*	−3·02**	5·53*	−4·27**
Religious denomination[b]	3·97*	2·28**	1·49^{ns}	1·07^{ns}
Familiarity with mental health care[a]	−9·23*	8·25*	−10·09*	8·72*

[a] Tested by t-statistic.   [b] Tested by F-statistic.
* Significant at the 0·001 level.   ** Significant at the 0·01 level.
^{ns} Not significant at the 0·05 level.

dependent variable was entered into the equation assuming that it satisfied conditions for entry based on the partial regression coefficient. Variables not contributing to the equation at or beyond the $0 \cdot 05$ significance level were excluded.

The results (table 7.6) show relatively low values of R^2 for each equation, indicating a small percentage of variation in beliefs explained by the linear combinations of personal characteristics. The values of R^2 range from a high of $0 \cdot 221$ (22%) for social restrictiveness to a low of $0 \cdot 150$ (15%) for benevolence. Two possible reasons for the weak explanatory power of the equations are: first, the inherent difficulty of predicting scores on abstract hypothetical constructs such as beliefs about the mentally ill; and, second, the limited set of independent variables used, in particular the proxy personality measures, are very restricted. This is not to suggest, however, that had a more comprehensive set of measures been available the values of R^2 would have increased dramatically. Variation in beliefs is typically elusive, not least because of the vulnerability of belief measures to error variance even in cases where considerable care has been taken in constructing and developing belief scales.

Considering the results in terms of the relative contribution of the independent variables to the equations shows that two variables (education level and familiarity with mental health care) are significant beyond the $0 \cdot 001$ level in each of the four equations. A third variable (church attendance) is as powerful except in the equation for benevolence. In contrast, number of children six to eighteen years of age enters only one equation—for CMHI—and then is the last variable to enter, only marginally exceeding the required $0 \cdot 05$ significance level. A second demographic

Table 7.6. Regression analysis results.

Independent variables	Dependent variable			
	authoritarianism	benevolence	social restrictiveness	CMHI
Age	ns	$-0 \cdot 21$ ***	$0 \cdot 062$ *	$-0 \cdot 033$ **
Sex	$-8 \cdot 78$ **	$1 \cdot 268$ *	ns	$1 \cdot 078$ **
Children (6–18)	ns	ns	ns	$-0 \cdot 479$ ***
Education	$-0 \cdot 911$ *	$0 \cdot 527$ *	$-0 \cdot 604$ *	$0 \cdot 475$ *
Tenure	ns	$-0 \cdot 785$ **	$0 \cdot 778$ ***	$-1 \cdot 858$ *
Church attendance	$-1 \cdot 546$ *	$0 \cdot 646$ ***	$-1 \cdot 324$ *	$1 \cdot 294$ *
Familiarity	$2 \cdot 285$ *	$-1 \cdot 972$ *	$2 \cdot 614$ *	$-2 \cdot 736$ *
Constant	$31 \cdot 530$ *	$21 \cdot 907$ *	$39 \cdot 884$ *	$20 \cdot 612$ *
R^2	$0 \cdot 217$	$0 \cdot 150$	$0 \cdot 221$	$0 \cdot 164$
Standard error of the estimate	$4 \cdot 532$	$4 \cdot 526$	$4 \cdot 897$	$5 \cdot 888$

* Significant at the $0 \cdot 001$ level.   ** Significant at the $0 \cdot 01$ level.
*** Significant at the $0 \cdot 05$ level.   ns Not significant at the $0 \cdot 05$ level.

variable, age, is also comparatively weak particularly as a predictor of authoritarianism and benevolence. Tenure status is similarly weak in two of the four equations, in this case authoritarianism and social restrictiveness. Finally, sex emerges as a moderate to strong predictor in three of the four equations, the exception being for social restrictiveness where it does not enter.

Overall, the regression results confirm the hypothesized links within the theoretical model even though the explained variance is relatively low for all four scales. In each of the four equations, demographic, socioeconomic, church attendance, and familiarity measures appear as significant predictors of beliefs about the mentally ill which can therefore be assumed at least in part to be a function of these broad types of population characteristics. These findings largely confirm the relationships reported in previous studies (see chapter 4), but go beyond them in that a more comprehensive range of personal characteristics has been examined in this analysis. In addition, their combined as well as separate effects on beliefs about the mentally ill have been tested.

7.2 Beliefs and attitudes

Following on from the link between external variables and beliefs, the next major relationship in the theoretical model is between beliefs and attitudes toward mental health facilities. Each of the three sets of beliefs are thought to influence attitudes and their effects will be discussed separately in this section beginning with the effects of beliefs about facility impacts.

7.2.1 Beliefs about facility impacts and attitudes toward facilities

For this analysis beliefs about facility impacts were measured in terms of the single composite scale described in the previous section. Attitudes toward facilities are based on the ratings of facility desirability for locations at three different distances from the respondent's home: seven to twelve blocks; two to six blocks; and within one block. Both measures are assumed to have interval-level properties and the relationships are tested by means of Pearson's correlation. The results (table 7.7) show strong correlations between the impact scale and each of the three desirability scales.

Table 7.7. Beliefs about facility impacts and attitudes to facilities[a].

Attitudes to facility	Composite belief scale
7 to 12 blocks	0·40
2 to 6 blocks	0·49
Within 1 block	0·52

[a] Figures are Pearson correlation coefficients, and all coefficients are significant beyond the 0·001 level.

The positive sign of the coefficients confirms the expected direction of the relationships. Those holding more negative beliefs about facility impacts express the more negative attitudes. The coefficients noticeably strengthen with decreasing distance for the desirability ratings, from 0·40 for the rating for a distance of seven to twelve blocks, to 0·52 for the rating for a distance of within one block. Later results involving these same attitude scales show a similar trend. The most likely explanation for this is that the variation in desirability ratings becomes increasingly systematic as the distance between facility and residence decreases. In other words, respondents are able to give more precise judgements of their attitudes for situations which most closely impinge upon them. The direction and strength of these relationships clearly confirms the link in the model between beliefs about facility impacts and attitudes toward facilities.

7.2.2 Beliefs about the mentally ill and attitudes toward facilities

The general hypothesis that attitudes to facilities are related to beliefs about the mentally ill was tested first by correlating scores on the four belief scales with the facility desirability ratings for the three distance zones. The correlations (table 7.8) show highly significant relationships between all four scales and the three separate desirability ratings. Considered by belief scale, the highest coefficients occur for the CMHI scale. This is the scale most directly concerned with community mental health, and it would therefore be expected to show the strongest correlation with the judged desirability of having a mental health facility located in the neighbourhood. The positive sign of the coefficients for CMHI is consistent with the hypothesis that facility locations will be judged more desirable by those expressing pro-CMHI sentiments.

After CMHI, the scale most strongly correlated with the desirability ratings is social restrictiveness. This scale expresses the view that the mentally ill pose a threat to society and that their activities should therefore be closely controlled and supervised. Those holding a prosocial

Table 7.8. Beliefs about the mentally ill and attitudes toward facilities[a]. (Source: Taylor and Dear, 1981, page 236.)

Scale	Distance zone		
	7–12 blocks	2–6 blocks	<1 block
Authoritarianism	−0·28	−0·36	−0·40
Benevolence	0·33	0·36	0·40
Social restrictiveness	−0·34	−0·44	−0·48
CMHI	0·45	0·57	0·61

[a] Pearson correlation coefficients, and all coefficients are significant beyond the 0·001 level.

restrictiveness view would be predicted as judging neighbourhood mental health facilities as undesirable and this is confirmed by the negative signs of the coefficients. The coefficients for authoritarianism and benevolence are slightly lower, but their signs confirm the working hypotheses. Pro-authoritarian views are associated with less favourable ratings of facilities and probenevolent sentiments coincide with more favourable ratings.

Considered by distance zone, the correlations show the same consistent pattern previously noted. For each scale the coefficients increase with decreasing distance.

A second test of the relationship between beliefs about the mentally ill and attitudes to facilities was performed by use of data obtained from the 139 respondents aware of an existing facility. These respondents were asked whether they were in favour, opposed, or indifferent towards the facility. A total of 95 reported being in favour, 19 were indifferent, and only 18 (13%) were opposed. A further test of the relationship between beliefs and attitudes is to determine how accurately these reactions to existing facilities can be predicted from beliefs about the mentally ill. A discriminant analysis was performed to assess this. Discriminant analysis determines how accurately membership in groups corresponding to categories of the dependent variable (in this case, in favour, opposed, and indifferent attitudes toward a facility) can be predicted from scores on a set of independent variables (here, scores on the four beliefs about the mentally ill scales). This involves the calculation of linear equations (discriminant functions) which maximally discriminate between the groups.

The results show first (table 7.9) that the mean scores on each of the belief scales are significantly different for the three groups defined on the basis of their attitudes to the existing facility (that is, in favour, indifferent, opposed). Moreover, the ordering of the group means show that the differences are in the hypothesized direction. Those opposed to the facility are the most authoritarian and socially restrictive and the least benevolent and community mental health oriented. In contrast, those in

Table 7.9. Beliefs about the mentally ill and attitudes to existing facilities[a]. (Source: Taylor et al, 1979, page 287.)

Scale	Reaction to facility[b]
Authoritarianism	$8 \cdot 56$ $(2 > 3 > 1)$
Benevolence	$9 \cdot 81$ $(1 > 3 > 2)$
Social restrictiveness	$12 \cdot 94$ $(2 > 3 > 1)$
CMHI	$21 \cdot 94$ $(1 > 3 > 2)$

[a] Analysis is based on number of respondents aware of a facility in their neighbourhood ($N = 139$), and the figures are F-statistics (F probability $< 0 \cdot 001$).
[b] 1 favour; 2 oppose; 3 indifferent.

favour of the facility were the least authoritarian and socially restrictive and the most benevolent and community mental health oriented. Consistently, the mean scores for the indifferent group lie between those for the other two groups on all four scales. Treating the scales in combination defines two discriminant functions. The discriminant function coefficients (table 7.10) indicate the relative contribution of the four scales to the discriminant equations. In the case of the first and most powerful function, the CMHI scale is the primary discriminating variable. For the second function it is the benevolence scale. The importance of the CMHI scale adds further support for its predictive validity.

A further capability of discriminant analysis is to calculate scores for each respondent on each of the discriminant functions. From these, a centroid score is derived for each group and respondents classified in terms of their proximity to the centroids. It is then possible to compare the predicted and actual group membership as a measure of the accuracy with which the scales in combination discriminate among the groups. The resulting contingency table (table 7.11) shows that overall 65% of cases were correctly classified. The associated chi-squared statistic is highly significant.

Table 7.10. Discriminant function coefficients for belief scales. (Source: Taylor et al, 1979, page 288.)

Scale	Function 1	Function 2
Authoritarianism	0·21	−1·00
Benevolence	0·29	−1·35
Social restrictiveness	0·05	−0·83
CMHI	1·15	−0·36

Table 7.11. Prediction of attitudes to existing facilities—with and without indifferent group included in the analysis; and all figures expressed as percentages. (Source: Taylor et al, 1979, page 288.)

Actual response	Predicted response [a]		
	favour	oppose	indifferent
Favour (95)	65	17	18
Oppose (18)	17	72	11
Indifferent (19)	16	21	63
	Predicted response [b]		
	favour	oppose	
Favour (95)	79	21	
Oppose (18)	22	78	

[a] 65% of all cases correctly classified: $\chi^2 = 63·03$ (significant beyond the 0·001 level).
[b] 79% of all cases correctly classified: $\chi^2 = 37·39$ (significant beyond the 0·001 level).

In percentage terms, those in the opposed group were most accurately predicted (72%), followed by those in favour (65%) and those indifferent (63%). This is a reasonable result given that we would expect the indifferent group to be less clearly identifiable than either of the extremes. The percentage of cases correctly classified is increased by omitting the indifferent group from the analysis. When this was done, 79% of total cases were correctly classified with 79% of those in favour accurately predicted and 78% of those opposed.

Considered overall, the results of the discriminant analysis provide further support for the general hypothesis that attitudes to facilities are related to beliefs about the mentally ill. More specifically, the four scales emerge as reasonably accurate predictors of attitudes toward existing facilities. The predictive validity of all four scales is therefore reinforced, although the strongest validation is clearly for the CMHI scale.

7.2.3 Beliefs about the neighbourhood and attitudes to facilities

Beliefs about the neighbourhood were measured by use of the seventy-eight-item adjective check list. Beliefs about facility characteristics were measured by use of the same check list. Comparison of the two sets of information provides a measure of congruence between facility and neighbourhood characteristics. On this basis it is possible to operationalize the theoretical concept of fit between form (the facility) and context (the neighbourhood) which in chapter 2 we suggested is likely to have an important influence on residents' attitudes to facilities. Fit essentially represents beliefs about the suitability of the neighbourhood as a location for a mental health facility. For this analysis, a derived measure of perceived fit between facility and neighbourhood is regarded as a more appropriate belief variable than any simple direct measure of neighbourhood beliefs.

Perceived fit was calculated as the differences between the adjective check list responses for the mental health facility and the neighbourhood on each of the six composite scales represented by the activity, evaluation, safety, integration, design, and predictability scales. Perceived fit was calculated by taking the difference between the standard score (see chapter 6) for the facility and for the neighbourhood on each scale. A negative scale score indicated that perception of the facility was not as positive as perception of the neighbourhood. A score of zero indicated correspondence between facility and neighbourhood perceptions for the particular scale. A positive scale score represented a more positive perception of the facility than of the neighbourhood.

The relationship between beliefs about the suitability of the neighbourhood as a location for a mental health facility and attitudes toward facilities was tested by correlating the perceived fit scores on each of the six scales with the desirability rating for a facility location within one block. The attitude measure was limited to the within-one-block rating because previous analysis had shown this to be the strongest correlate of beliefs. The correlations (table 7.12) show highly significant relationships between all six scales and facility desirability, although the coefficients themselves are relatively low. The positive direction of the relationships supports the hypothesis that facility desirability is directly related to beliefs about the suitability of the neighbourhood as a location for a facility. Of the six scales, the strongest relationships are with the evaluation, design, and integration scales with weaker relationships for the safety, predictability, and activity scales. This ordering makes intuitive sense in that the more clearly evaluative scales tend to show the stronger relationships.

Although the relationships shown by this analysis are relatively weak, the hypothesis linking beliefs about the neighbourhood with attitudes to facilities is confirmed. It is hardly surprising that the relationships are weak because of the inherent complexity of obtaining satisfactory empirical measures of such an intangible hypothetical concept as perceived fit. Our use of the adjective check list scales to this end represents a novel approach to the problem. We consider that these results justify further applications of the scales in similar future studies.

Taken together, the results presented in this section provide strong support for the links between beliefs and attitudes contained in the theoretical model. Of the three sets of beliefs considered, beliefs about the mentally ill show the strongest relationships with attitudes to facilities. This probably reflects two factors, one substantive and the other methodological. The first is the importance of beliefs about the users of facilities in shaping attitudes to the facilities themselves. We suggested in chapter 2, in discussing the model, that individual and community response to facilities is almost certainly more a response to the user than to the facility and the empirical findings support this assertion. The second factor which possibly contributes to the strength of the relationships for the beliefs about the mentally ill scales is the methodological refinement of the measures. As described in chapter 6, considerable effort was expended to develop reliable and valid scales capable of providing precise measures

Table 7.12. Beliefs about neighbourhood–facility fit and attitudes to facilities[a].

Perceived fit scales	Attitude to facility within one block
Activity	0·07
Evaluation	0·14
Safety	0·11
Integration	0·13
Design	0·14
Predictability	0·08

[a] Figures are Kendall's tau correlation coefficients, all coefficients significant beyond the 0·001 level.

of beliefs. The predictive validity of the scales demonstrated in this analysis confirms their methodological strength. We hope that future applications will lead to their further refinement.

7.3 Attitudes and behavioural intentions

The third major link within the theoretical model that the Toronto data allow us to test is that between attitudes to facilities and behavioural intentions. For this analysis, the facility desirability ratings for the three distance zones formed the attitude measures. Behavioural intentions were recorded in the questionnaire by asking each respondent to indicate which of nine listed actions he or she was most likely to take in opposition to facility locations previously rated to some degree undesirable. The nine actions (table 7.13) were grouped into four categories prior to analysis: oppose and do nothing, oppose and intend group action, oppose and intend individual action, oppose and consider moving. In this order the categories represent an ordinal scale of increasing opposition. In the analysis this index of behavioural intentions was treated as both nominal and ordinal.

Two important implications follow from the way in which the information on behavioural intentions was obtained. Since the question was only asked of those who had previously rated a facility location undesirable, the attitude and behavioural intentions measured are necessarily non-independent. A valid test of the relationship, therefore, has to be restricted to those respondents who rated the facility locations undesirable. The hypothesis then is that behavioural intentions vary with the degree of undesirability expressed. The second implication is that the number of respondents for the analysis differs for each of the three facility distance zones. Of the total sample of 1090, 128 gave ratings to some degree undesirable for the seven-to-twelve block zone; 255 for the two-to-six block zone; and 404 for the within-one-block zone. This sequence confirms that the nearer the potential location is to home the more likely it will be rated as undesirable (see chapter 8 for further discussion).

Figure 7.13. Behavioural intentions index.

Category	Actions
Intend no action	oppose and do nothing
Intend group action	oppose and sign petition
	oppose and attend meeting
	oppose and join protest group
	oppose and form protest group
Intend individual action	oppose and write to newspaper
	oppose and contact politician
	oppose and contact other government official
Consider moving	oppose and consider moving

It is revealing, however, that even for locations within one block of home, 63% of respondents gave neutral or desirable ratings.

In the first analysis, the behavioural intentions index was treated as nominal and a Kruskal–Wallis analysis of variance was performed to test for significant differences in the undesirability ratings among the four groups defined by the index. Three tests were conducted, one for each distance zone. The results (table 7.14) show highly significant differences in two of the three tests, the exception being for the seven-to-twelve-block zone where the result is not significant. As with previous results, we see that the relationship strengthens with decreasing distance to home, again implying greater systematic variance in the data for these judgements. The mean ranks for each group indicate the direction of the differences for the two significant tests. In both cases, the mean rank increases from group 1 (oppose and do nothing) to group 4 (oppose and consider moving), which shows that those who would do nothing gave on average the most positive ratings and those who would consider moving the least positive. This directionality confirms the ordering of the groups previously described

Table 7.14. Attitudes and behavioural intentions: results of a Kruskal–Wallis analysis of variance test.

	Behavioural intention groups				
	nothing	group action	individual action	move	χ^2
Distance zone: 7–12 blocks					
N	48	45	22	10	$5 \cdot 91$ [ns]
$\bar{R}$	$55 \cdot 13$	$64 \cdot 17$	$75 \cdot 18$	$68 \cdot 75$	
Distance zone: 2–6 blocks					
N	79	91	62	23	$38 \cdot 91$ [*]
$\bar{R}$	$88 \cdot 67$	$139 \cdot 67$	$144 \cdot 71$	$171 \cdot 87$	
Distance zone: <1 block					
N	121	97	98	86	$82 \cdot 80$ [*]
$\bar{R}$	$136 \cdot 92$	$203 \cdot 73$	$215 \cdot 18$	$274 \cdot 27$	

[*] Significant beyond the $0 \cdot 001$ level, [ns] not significant at the $0 \cdot 05$ level.

Table 7.15. Attitudes and behavioural intentions: rank-order correlations.

Distance zones	Rank correlations	Number of cases[a]
7–12 blocks	$0 \cdot 2070$ [***]	125
2–6 blocks	$0 \cdot 3653$ [*]	255
<1 block	$0 \cdot 4428$ [*]	402

[*] Significant beyond the $0 \cdot 001$ level.   [***] Significant beyond the $0 \cdot 05$ level.
[a] Number of missing cases = 50.

and leads on to the second set of tests which assumes ordinal properties for the behavioural intentions index.

For the second set of tests, Spearman rank-order correlations were calculated. The results (table 7.15) show significant positive correlations confirming a direct relationship between the undesirability of a facility and the strength of behavioural intentions. Once again there is a clear strengthening of the relationship with decreasing distance to home. Taken together the two sets of results provide strong support for the link between attitudes and behavioural intentions in the theoretical model. The more negative a person's attitude toward a facility the more likely he or she will take action to oppose it. Furthermore, the more negative the attitude the more likely the action will involve a strong personal commitment, either to some form of individual protest or to a consideration of moving out of the neighbourhood.

7.4 Behaviour and outcomes
The results of the analysis based on the Toronto data have shown strong support for the links between four of the major components in the theoretical model, namely the links between external variables and beliefs, between beliefs and attitudes, and between attitudes and behavioural intentions. The final major relationship, between behavioural intentions and actual behaviour, cannot be tested by means of the Toronto data because so few respondents reported having taken any action in response to a facility. In chapter 2 we discussed the potential problems involved in measuring behaviour and observed that, within a general population sample, it was quite likely that very few respondents would have undertaken any of the behaviours of interest. In the sample design, we attempted to circumvent this problem by purposely selecting one group of respondents ($N = 388$) from areas with existing facilities. In this way we were ensuring that a substantial number of respondents had facilities close to their home and therefore potentially had reason for engaging in action.

Somewhat surprisingly, however, we found a relatively low level of facility awareness. Only 83 of the 388 respondents living within a quarter mile of existing facilities were aware of their presence, and of these 83 only 33 could correctly identify the facility by name and location. An additional 56 respondents in the without facilities sample indicated awareness of a facility in their neighbourhood because of the subjective definition of neighbourhood. Adding these 56 to the 83 from the with facilities sample gives a maximum of 139 respondents aware of a facility and therefore likely to have taken any action. But, in fact, of those aware only 18 were opposed to the facility and only 5 of them had actually taken any action in opposition. Clearly, these numbers are far too small to permit any statistical analysis of the relationship with behaviour.

The strength of the relationship between behavioural intentions and behaviour therefore remains undetermined. In fact, it is difficult to conceive how this relationship could be satisfactorily investigated by means of cross-sectional data. Ideally, a longitudinal study is required providing, for example, information on behavioural intentions prior to any proposal to locate a facility in a neighbourhood and subsequently information on actual behaviour during such time that a proposal is under review and, if relevant, during a specified period after facility opening. We intend in a follow-up to the Toronto study to attempt such an investigation.

An important question is whether the small number of active opponents to local mental health facilities in the Toronto sample accurately reflects response in the population at large. We are confident that it does, despite the fact that it seems counter to the common impression that mental health facilities are generally unwanted and generate widespread community opposition. We base our conclusion on our data being drawn from rigorous, stratified random samples. A valid comment on the data is that they do not represent the reactions of residents either immediately prior to, or following, the location of a facility in their neighbourhood. This is the stage when opposition is usually most evident, and the lack of such time-specific data may partly account for the generally positive responses observed. It remains difficult, however, to account for the low level of awareness of existing facilities even if allowance is made for their general unobtrusiveness. Had the opening of a facility resulted in widespread opposition, we would expect at least a general awareness of its existence, unless we are willing to assume that many of the present residents moved into the neighbourhood after the opening. Moreover, the general level of recent public debate in Toronto over the location of residential facilities for the socially, mentally, and physically disabled has been very high. It is equally difficult to account for the large majority of responses in favour of existing facilities, unless we assume a major shift in opinion in light of experience of the facility's operation and effect on the neighbourhood. None of these alternative explanations seems very convincing. We conclude, therefore, that in Toronto active opposition to neighbourhood mental health facilities is probably limited in many instances to a small vocal minority whose views are not representative of their community as a whole.

We should not, however, underestimate the influence that this small minority of opponents can exert. Nor can we conclude that facility acceptance will be the normal outcome of decisions to locate facilities in local neighbourhoods. The reasons for this were referred to in chapter 2 in discussing the link between behaviour and outcomes. Facility acceptance or rejection is normally the product of group rather than individual action. Extraneous group-based factors, especially the political power and influence vested in particular social groups, complicate the link between individual behaviour and outcomes. It follows that a small, but powerful, minority can succeed in opposing a facility location. This is most likely to occur when a substantial proportion of the nonopponents take a neutral stance such that there is little, if any, active public support for a facility.

Under these circumstances the views of the vocal minority are quite likely to be decisive because the silent majority remains silent. In this regard, note that in the Toronto sample over 30% indicated neutral views based on the facility desirability ratings. Therefore, the level of support for facilities may well be more apparent than real and may well have little bearing on the outcomes of decisions to locate facilities in residential neighbourhoods. Without investigating the dynamics of particular controversies over facility locations, we can only speculate on the link between behaviour and outcomes. However, recent events in Toronto support the view that the small, vocal minority of opponents can have a far greater influence on the facility location process than the silent majority comprising those who are either neutral or in principle supporters of facilities. In short, the generally positive response shown by the Toronto study and the level of opposition evident in recent controversies over facilities in Toronto and elsewhere are by no means irreconcilable.

7.5 Conclusions

The analysis presented in this chapter provides a direct test of the theoretical model proposed in chapter 2. The model is supported. The Toronto study data confirm the relationships between external variables and beliefs, between beliefs and attitudes, and between attitudes and behavioural intentions.

The links between external variables and beliefs is confirmed by the significant, though weak, relationships between facility awareness and beliefs about facility impacts. Stronger relationships were found between a range of personal characteristics and beliefs about facility impacts and also beliefs about the mentally ill. With regard to the latter, these results are an important advance on those previously reported in that a wider range of personal characteristics are treated and their joint as well as their separate effects are examined. The link between beliefs and attitudes was confirmed for all three sets of beliefs. The strongest relationships were for beliefs about the mentally ill, supporting the view that attitudes to facilities are primarily a response to the users. Attitudes and behavioural intentions were strongly related. Those rating facilities as more undesirable are more likely to intend an action in opposition. Furthermore, the degree of commitment to individual action is directly related to the strength of negative attitudes.

The Toronto data do not allow a test of the relationship between behavioural intentions and behaviour because too few respondents had actually taken any action. This was despite the fact that approximately one third of the sample was drawn from areas with existing facilities. The implication of this low level of behavioural response and the generally positive or neutral opinions expressed about facilities is that active opposition is limited to a small vocal minority. We caution, however, against the conclusion that, because of this limited opposition, facility locations will meet with easy acceptance in the community. We recognize that the opponents, though in the minority, can determine community response to facilities if they have political power and influence and if the nonopponents remain silent and voice no clear support.

We have chosen in presenting this analysis to deal with each set of relationships separately. A logical next step is to construct an analytical model which would examine these relationships simultaneously. This would allow a more precise estimation of the degree of interaction among the variables and an assessment of the overall power of the model to explain and to predict attitudinal and behavioural responses to facilities. Causal analysis provides a potential tool for doing this. The development and testing of a causal model for the Toronto study lies beyond the scope of this book, but it is the focus of work in progress, and interested readers are referred to Hall (1980).

In summary, this analysis shows that behavioural intentions toward neighbourhood mental health facilities are a product of residents' attitudes. In turn, these attitudes are a function of various sets of beliefs including beliefs about facility impacts, about the mentally ill, and about the suitability of the neighbourhood as a facility location. Moreover, individual beliefs can be related back to a range of external variables of which personal characteristics, including socioeconomic status, church attendance, and familiarity with the mentally ill, are the strongest correlates. These results add significantly to our understanding of the factors affecting individual attitudinal and behavioural responses to facilities. At the same time, in more general terms, they provide further support for the Fishbein–Ajzen theory of reasoned action which is the basis for our theoretical model.

Part 5: Neighbourhood impacts of mental health facilities

8 External effects of mental health facilities

This is the first of two chapters in which we examine our second major empirical objective, the neighbourhood impacts of mental health facilities. Attention focusses on the spatial externalities associated with these facilities. In this chapter we use the Toronto survey data to determine external effects as perceived by local residents. In the following chapter, real estate data for Metropolitan Toronto are the basis for analyzing the effect of facility locations on property values, an effect which is commonly feared, although to date empirically unsubstantiated.

The existence and importance of externalities in urban areas has long been conceded. Externalities in production are one reason why cities exist, whereas externalities in consumption are a significant force for residential differentiation. However, research on the spatial incidence of external effects is less well-developed. In spite of recent attempts to clarify the theoretical bases of spatial externalities, little is known about their existence and incidence in the real world (Papageorgiou, 1978). Moreover, the extent and nature of the behavioural responses which spatial externalities induce in the impacted population are scarcely mentioned.

In this chapter, therefore, we proceed with a dual concern. First, it seems important to illuminate the nature of the external effects associated with community-based mental health facilities. Second, it is necessary to place a further perspective on the precise role of externalities in the construction of urban space, by examining the nature of the behavioural response to the incidence of such externalities. To address these issues, the chapter reviews the role of spatial externalities in community mental health, and generates three specific research analyses regarding the nature, spatial extent of, and behavioural response to external effects.

8.1 Spatial externalities and community mental health facilities
The mere presence of an external effect is of little interest unless it can be shown to have demonstrable consequences for human welfare or environmental quality. However, when such consequences are in evidence, the incidence of externalities is a potent force for conflict. An extended sequence of fractious political dispute is usually involved (Harvey, 1973, chapter 2). Often, a judgement has to be made between direct service benefits and externality costs; for instance, the benefits of a nearby fire station may typically offset the nuisance of constant vehicular traffic. The cataclysmic impact of externality effects is an important element in Papageorgiou's recent characterization of the urban landscape. He suggests that urban form is a product of two unfolding surfaces: a 'population surface' and an 'externality surface'. The exact structure of the externality source determines the nature of the interaction between the two surfaces and hence, the concomitant urban form (Papageorgiou, 1978).

The behavioural response to an externality field appears to be a function of the threat imposed by that field. The greater the potential disruption promised by the external effects, the more intense is the community response. It is important to recognize that individuals and groups have different 'stakes' in their daily-life environments (Olives, 1976). A resource-rich, middle-class neighbourhood is likely to be defended from encroachment more vociferously than a transient, resource-deficient area (Peet, 1975). Thus, it may be possible to observe a different behavioural response to an identical externality source according to each subpopulation's attitudinal predisposition (see chapter 7). Such a response is then recorded as an adjustment to the prior pattern in the population surface.

Recent analyses have focussed attention on three dimensions of the spatial externality field: its intensity, extent, and rate of distance decay (figure 8.1). The intensity of the externality field provides a measure of the total impact of the externality source in its immediate vicinity. It could be measured, for instance, in terms of property value decline, or noise levels. The extent of the field refers to the absolute geographical area covered by the external effect. This is, of course, linked to the rate of distance decay in the externality impact, which summarizes the rate at which the external effect dissipates over space.

The dimensions of an externality field associated with any facility will vary according to the scale, type, number, and degree of noxiousness of the facility in question (Dear, 1976). For example, ceteris paribus the

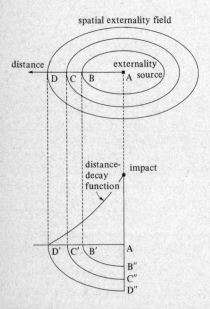

Figure 8.1. Dimensions of the spatial externality field. (Source: Dear et al, 1980, page 344.)

larger the facility the greater its potential impact. However, the precise impact of any externality source will also depend upon the characteristics of the population surface with which it intersects. Hence, it has been shown that community response to externalities will vary with the socio-economic structure of neighbourhoods (Taylor and Hall, 1977), as well as with the physical characteristics of the neighbourhood, including land-use mix and density of development.

For present purposes, the externality source is the community mental health facility itself. Extensive media coverage seems to confirm the notion that mental health facilities are considered as 'noxious', that is, they are needed within a given area, but not desired (for whatever reason) by residents adjacent to a potential site. In general terms, the existence and significance of nonuser, neighbourhood-associated external effects in association with community mental health facilities has not been widely researched. However, previous research has suggested that behavioural response is determined largely by community predispositions toward the mentally ill (Rabkin, 1974; Segal, 1978). The mental health facility may or may not be a compounding factor in the resultant behavioural response.

In contrast with the wealth of literature on community attitudes toward the mentally ill (see chapter 4), very little research has been undertaken to ascertain the relevant dimensions of community attitudes toward mental health facilities. In general terms, a distinction has been made between the tangible and intangible external effects of a facility (Dear et al, 1977). The former are those which are readily quantifiable, such as the potential effect of facilities on neighbourhood property values or on traffic generation. The latter externalities refer to the nonquantifiable sources of community opposition, such as fear for personal security or property. However, the structural characteristics of a facility itself are also important in generating community opposition, including the facility's design, attractiveness, and condition (Western Institute for Research in Mental Health, 1967). In another study, Thouez suggested that community attitudes toward public facilities could be measured along the more abstract dimensions of evaluation, activity, strength, and familiarity (Thouez, 1975).

Other reports, from a diverse literature, have emphasized the user-associated external effects of mental health facilities. They include, for instance, assessments of the 'invisible' support network provided for ex-patients by community resources (Gonen, 1977; Segal and Aviram, 1978; Smith, 1976b); and examinations of the unanticipated spillover effects of the shift to community-based mental health care, including changes in the fiscal burden (Scull, 1978; Wolpert and Wolpert, 1976). In addition, an increasing literature is developing on the 'colocational' patterns of different sets of human service facilities. For example, White (1979) has shown that a high degree of locational interdependency exists in metropolitan areas among facilities for the mentally ill, the mentally retarded, and other service-dependent groups. Wolch (1979; 1980) has also demonstrated the logic of the residential location behaviour which leads to a concentration of service-dependent populations in the inner city (see Chapter 2).

In light of the complexity of this problem, and the relative dearth of information, the objectives of this chapter are modest and direct. We wish to establish the fundamental dimensions of the spatial externality field associated with community mental health facilities. Three specific research objectives may be identified:
(1) to identify the *nature* of the externality effects associated with community mental health facilities, as perceived by the 'host' community;
(2) to demonstrate the *spatial extent* of the externality field; and
(3) to indicate the degree of *behavioural response* which may be anticipated as a consequence of the externality field.

8.2 The external effects of mental health facilities
In light of the media-reported opposition to community mental health facility locations, it would be folly to deny the existence of an associated externality effect. However, as we have seen, very little systematic evidence exists on the real-world incidence of such externalities. A fundamental point of departure, therefore, is to determine the dimensions of the externality surface associated with mental health facilities.

In free response to an open-ended question, all respondents were asked to assess the potential impact of a community mental health facility. Almost one-third of the sample anticipated little or no effect, although another 27% viewed a facility positively (table 8.1). This latter group seemed strongly motivated by the direct service benefits associated with a facility. On the other hand, less than one-quarter of the respondents considered that a facility might have a negative impact. Specific reasons for this attitude were diverse, but a small minority (7%) found the situation

Table 8.1. Neighbourhood impact of mental health facility location (percentage frequency: $N = 1090$). (Source: Dear et al, 1980, page 347.)

Negative impact:		Little or no effect	31
bad	7		
bad, if no client supervision	0	Positive impact:	
bad, depending on type of client	0	good	12
bad, if too close	1	good, if client supervision	2
likely to generate opposition	3	good, depending on type of client	1
bring undesirable people in	1	good, if not too close	1
reduce land values	2	helpful to community residents	11
threatening	2	upgrade neighbourhood	0
arouse community fear	5	Subtotal—positive impact	27
increase crime	0		
increase noise	1	Other	4
depress community residents	1	Do not know, no response	14
give area a bad name	1		
Subtotal—negative impact	24	Total	100

threatening or fear-arousing. This finding is consistent with others which have stressed residents' fears about the potential unpredictability and dangerousness of mental patients.

Respondents' ratings of a facility on twelve bipolar impact scales provided a more structured measure of anticipated externality effects. These ratings were described in the preceding chapter where they functioned as measures of beliefs about facility impacts and hence only a brief summary of the results is necessary here. Ratings were on a seven-point scale with three scale-points corresponding to positive impacts, three to negative impacts, and one neutral midpoint. The scale was reduced to three points (positive, neutral, and negative), and only the percentage of total responses in each category is reported (table 7.1). The responses of those aware and unaware of a facility in their neighbourhood are distinguished.

The pattern of response for the unaware group shows a modal response of neutral for all twelve impact scales, with the percentages ranging from 39% on the *resident satisfaction* scale to 64% on the *property taxes* scale. The percentage of negative ratings exceeds the percentage of positive ratings on all twelve scales, the difference being greatest on the *property values* and *traffic volume* scales. The popular perception that locating mental health facilities in residential neighbourhoods has a detrimental effect on property values is reflected in these results. However, the generally benign expectations of the respondents are consistent with the free responses (table 8.1).

The percentage distributions for the aware group indicate in general that direct experience of the neighbourhood impact of community mental health facilities results in less negative perceptions. The modal response is again neutral for all twelve scales and, with only one exception, the percentages are higher than for the unaware subsample. For two scales (*residential character and property taxes*) the percentage of positive responses is greater than the percentage negative. For the remaining ten impacts the percentage of negative responses exceeds the percentage positive, but compared with the results for the unaware group the difference is in general reduced. An exception is the *property value* scale, where the difference in positive and negative responses for the two groups is equal. [This is an intriguing result because we shall see (in chapter 9) that, for a subset of the neighbourhoods included in the study, mental health facilities had little or no measurable effect on property values. Nonetheless, they still seem to be perceived to have a detrimental effect.]

Overall, the preponderance of neutral responses both for the aware and for the unaware groups indicates the extent of indifference to, and ignorance of, the neighbourhood impacts of mental health facilities. Since in almost all cases the negative perceptions exceed the positive, there is more likely to be opposition than support for a facility. At the same time, however, the apparent 'softening' of opinion with awareness and

knowledge of the effects of a facility suggests that the anticipated impacts
are worse than those actually experienced.

8.3 Spatial extent of the externality field

Whatever the precise nature of the externality effect, its impact is likely to
be experienced over a limited spatial field, and its most intense impact
to be felt nearest the externality source. Thus, what is of interest is the
spatial extent and intensity of the externality field, and its rate of decay
with increased distance from the source. As we have seen, the rate of
distance decay will vary with several factors, notably the scale or type of
facility, and the structure of the host community. In this section, we
examine the limits of the externality field associated with mental health
facilities, and how various facility types may alter the form of the field.

   Respondents were asked to rate the desirability of having a community
mental health facility within seven to twelve blocks, two to six blocks,
and less than one block from their homes. A nine-point scale was used,
with 9 representing extremely undesirable; 1, extremely desirable; and 5,
the neutral response (see chapter 5). The general pattern of responses
indicates a clear distance-decay effect in residents' attitudes (figure 8.2).
In spite of a strongly consistent 'neutral' core, the proportion of residents
rating a facility as to any extent undesirable diminishes from about 40%
(within one block) to 12% (at seven to twelve blocks). For further
analysis, the four negative and four positive responses are aggregated into

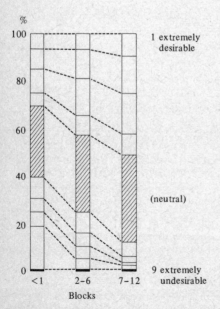

Figure 8.2. Distance-decay effect in facility desirability. (Source: Dear et al, 1980,
page 349.)

two general categories representing 'desirable' and 'undesirable' ratings (table 8.2). Responses vary in relation to proximity to facility and awareness/unawareness of a facility. At a distance of seven to twelve blocks, only a small minority rated a facility as undesirable. Those that were aware of a facility in their neighbourhood were apparently more tolerant than the unaware; over 50% of the sample viewed a facility as desirable. However, within one block of home, 40·6% of the unaware group regarded a facility as undesirable, and only 29·8% as desirable. Those aware of a specific facility express more positive attitudes toward facilities in general at this closest distance.

These trends are confirmed by a nonparametric analysis of variance (table 8.3). Simply stated, our sample group tends to respond as three distinct populations as proximity to a facility increases. This distinctiveness is preserved both in the aware and in the unaware groups. Although the direction of change is toward increasing undesirability as proximity increases, it is significant that (except in one instance) the median score for each subpopulation is less than 5, which implies an overall positive evaluation of community mental health facilities. The analysis also confirms that the aware and unaware groups are significantly different in

Table 8.2. Desirability of mental health facility by proximity to respondent's home (column percentages)[a]. (Source: Dear et al, 1980, page 349.)

| Response [b] | Distance zones | | | | | |
| | 7–12 blocks | | 2–6 blocks | | <1 block | |
	aware	unaware	aware	unaware	aware	unaware
Desirable	52·2	50·8	52·2	41·6	43·5	29·8
Neutral	36·8	37·1	33·1	32·8	30·9	29·6
Undesirable	11·1	12·1	14·6	25·4	25·7	40·6

[a] Aware of facility, $N = 136$; unaware, did not know of facility, $N = 938$.
[b] Number of missing cases = 16.

Table 8.3. Desirability of mental health facility by proximity to respondent's home (median scores). (Source: Dear et al, 1980, page 349.)

| Respondent subpopulations [a] | Distance zones | | | Friedman– Anova statistic (χ^2) |
	7–12 blocks	2–6 blocks	<1 block	
Aware ($N = 136$)	4·0	4·2	4·7	15·9 [**]
Not aware ($N = 938$)	4·4	4·8	4·1	361·5 [**]
χ^2	insignificant	16·342 [***]	19·420 [***]	

[**] Significant at less than the 0·01 level.   [***] Significant at less than the 0·05 level.
[b] Number of missing cases = 16.

their responses over the two inner-distance zones. Within six blocks of a facility, the aware group are significantly more tolerant (as indicated by their median scores and the Friedman analysis of variance). The absence of distinction between the aware and unaware groups beyond the six-block range suggests that distance from a facility is so great as to neutralize any perceptual differences between the two groups. This confirms our a priori notions on the spatially constrained nature of the externality field, and emphasizes the importance of the association between tolerance and facility awareness.

These results add to the continuing debate over the effects of familiarity with mental illness, and by extension mental health facilities, on public acceptance of patients and facilities. Smith and Hanham (1981) have recently reported the results of a study which indicate the need to distinguish between spatial and social proximity to the mentally ill. Their findings show a positive relationship between geographic proximity to a mental hospital and acceptance of patients, but an inverse relationship between acceptance and social proximity measured in terms of personal contact and acquaintance with the mentally ill. Our results on the effects of awareness imply that spatial proximity may engender more positive attitudes, but not to the extent reported by Smith and Hanham that the acceptance of facilities actually increases as distance from the facility decreases.

One major factor affecting the externality field is the exact nature of the externality source. To assess the effect of *type of facility* on the externality surface, a separate analysis of the desirability ratings was performed for the subsample who could identify the existing mental health facility in their neighbourhood (a total of 83 respondents out of the 388 originally selected because of the facility present in their locality). Respondents in this reduced sample lived in the vicinity of one of three types of facility: (1) *outpatient*, which provides services for the ambulatory mentally ill, much like a regular hospital-based outpatient unit; (2) *group home*, which provides permanent or semipermanent residential facilities for ex-patients; and (3) *social-therapeutic centres* which provide social, recreational, and counselling services on an inter- mittent basis.

The desirability ratings for the three subgroups (table 8.4) show that respondents living close to social-therapeutic facilities tend to rate mental health facilities in general more favourably than do those living near either of the other two facility types. (We reemphasize that respondents were not asked to rate their local facility, but rather the desirability of having a mental health facility of any kind located at the three different distances from their home.) The inference we draw from table 8.4 is that awareness of, and proximity to, a social-therapeutic facility has some positive effect on attitudes toward facilities in general. This is clearly seen by comparing the median ratings at each distance for the social- therapeutic group with the corresponding figures for the other two aware groups (table 8.4) and with the medians for the aware and unaware groups as a whole (table 8.3). We recognize, however, that the sample sizes for the three aware subgroups are relatively small and, as a consequence, a Kruskal–Wallis analysis of variance showed no statistically significant between-group differences in the ratings for any of the three distance zones. Nevertheless, taken together with the results previously discussed, there is some evidence, albeit tentative, to indicate that not only are the aware group in general more favourably disposed to mental health facilities, but also that, among those aware, residents are influenced in their attitudes by the particular type of facility which they know.

Table 8.4. Desirability of different facility types by proximity to resident's home (column percentages)[a]. (Source: Dear et al, 1980, page 350.)

Response	Distance zones and facility[b]								
	7–12 blocks			2–6 blocks			<1 block		
	OP	GH	ST	OP	GH	ST	OP	GH	ST
Desirable	47·8	46·8	66·7	47·8	49·0	66·7	39·1	40·3	58·3
Neutral	30·4	48·9	16·7	30·4	40·4	16·7	30·4	36·2	25·0
Undesirable	21·7	4·2	8·3	21·6	10·6	8·3	30·4	23·4	8·3
Median score	5·0	5·0	2·0	5·0	5·0	2·5	5·0	5·0	3·5

[a] Columns do not sum to 100 because of one missing value.
[b] OP—outpatient facility ($N = 23$); GH—group home ($N = 47$); ST—social-therapeutic facility ($N = 12$).

8.4 Spatial externality and behavioural response
Our theoretical preconceptions tend to suggest that the population surface is in a constant process of readjustment to the incidence of the externality surfaces in urban space. What is the nature of this readjustment in the case of mental health facilities? To assess the degree of behavioural response, the sample population who considered any facility–distance combination as undesirable were asked what action they would be likely to take in opposition. They were shown a list of nine possible options (table 8.5; also see chapter 7). The modal response of this reduced sample was 1 (do nothing). However, significant percentages of the population would also be willing to participate in some form of group action (categories 5 through 8), especially signing petitions. or attending meetings. Few acts of individual opposition are anticipated (categories 2 through 4, table 8.5). The most significant change in response behaviour over the three distance zones is in the final category (9)—consider moving. This proportion increases from 7·8% of the respondents in a range of seven to twelve blocks, to 21·6% in a range of less than one block range. This pattern of more intense response in closer proximity to a facility is

consistent with the observation that those with a greater 'stake' in an
environment will tend to react with greater intensity if that environment is
threatened (Olives, 1976). The pattern of behavioural intentions by those
aware of a facility in their neighbourhood did not differ significantly
from this general pattern, although it should be noted that the number in
this subsample is quite small (table 8.5, figures in parentheses).

   The evidence seems to indicate a potentially high level of neighbourhood
opposition activity amongst those who rate a facility as to some degree
undesirable. However, other survey evidence tends to contradict this
conclusion, and reemphasizes the complexity of the relationship between
intentions and actual behaviour discussed in an earlier chapter (see section
2.3.7). For example, only 9 of the 404 respondents in the unaware group
had actually taken any one of the actions in opposition to a community
facility. Moreover, of the 139 respondents aware of their local mental
health centre, only 18 were opposed to it, and only 5 of that 18 actively
opposed the location. One person had signed a petition, two had attended
a meeting, and one had considered moving. On the other hand, it may be
countered that our sample design underestimates the degree of actual
opposition, since it necessarily omitted those respondents whose opposition
was intense enough to cause them to leave the neighbourhood. Hence, we
are sampling only two out of a necessary three populations: those
responding to a hypothetical location, and those responding to an existing
location. A complete study would, of course, wish to sample from a
population in the throes of a locational controversy in order to gauge the
full extent of opposition. However, given the extremely small numbers in
opposition, and the difficulties of moving in a tight housing market, we

Table 8.5. Proposed action by opposition group by distance zone (column percentages)[a].
(Source: Dear et al, 1980, page 350.)

Behavioural response category	Distance zone		
	7–12 blocks	2–6 blocks	<1 block
1 Do nothing	39·1 (26·7)	31·0 (25·0)	30·2 (28·6)
2 Write to newspaper	0·8 (0·0)	2·0 (0·0)	2·2 (0·0)
3 Contact politician	7·8 (13·3)	8·2 (5·0)	6·4 (2·9)
4 Contact other government official	3·9 (0·0)	5·9 (5·0)	3·7 (5·7)
5 Sign petition	23·4 (46·7)	19·6 (25·0)	11·6 (17·1)
6 Attend meeting	10·2 (6·7)	15·7 (20·0)	14·4 (17·1)
7 Join protest group	4·7 (0·0)	6·3 (10·0)	5·7 (5·7)
8 Form protest group	2·3 (0·0)	2·4 (0·0)	4·2 (5·7)
9 Consider moving	7·8 (6·7)	9·9 (10·0)	21·6 (17·1)
Total	100·0 (100·0)	100·0 (100·0)	100·0 (100·0)
N	128 (15)	255 (20)	404 (35)

[a] Figures in parentheses indicate responses of those people aware of the facility existing
in their neighbourhood.

surmise that the number of people who have already exited in response to the facility location is likely to be negligible. In this case, therefore, we conclude that there have been only relatively minor adjustments in the population surface as a consequence of a new externality source (a community mental health facility).

8.5 Perception of external effects by various population subsamples

Our previous analysis (see chapter 7) has suggested that important variations in neighbourhood reaction to mental health facilities may be due to differences in social class, neighbourhood cohesion, etc. It therefore seemed important to try to determine the variation in response to perceived externality effects according to such factors. Accordingly, an exhaustive research design was constructed to take account of variations along five possible dimensions:
1. social status, characterized by low, middle, and upper income categories;
2. land-use mix, defined according to three major categories—single-family residential, multiple-family residential, and commercial/industrial;
3. facility type, which recognizes the fundamental difference between a group home (a residential facility) and a social-therapeutic/outpatient unit (characterized by short-term, intermittent visits);
4. neighbourhood saturation, describing the presence of more than one facility in a given neighbourhood; and
5. distance from a facility, according to straight-line and block-front measures, and intended to act as a surrogate for respondent 'stake' in the neighbourhood.

The results of these tests are not fully reported here, since difficulties in sample size prevented a consistent statistical analysis of variations along these five dimensions. The reader interested in the detailed results is referred to Boeckh (1980). Instead, we merely present a tabular summary of these findings, since the method and results will be of use to future researchers (table 8.6). It should also be pointed out that, although the results are not statistically significant, the pattern of results in the raw data is sufficiently suggestive to warrant a further investigation of this topic (see Boeckh, 1980, chapters 5 and 6). For the moment, we are content to observe that the four disaggregated variables (social status, land-use mix, facility type, and neighbourhood saturation) do not significantly alter the interpretation of respondent perceptions already reported in this chapter. For example, no significant variations are found in responses to anticipated externality effect (compare table 7.1), desirability of a proximate facility (table 8.2), or proposed behavioural response (table 8.5) because of the type of facility in a respondent's neighbourhood. The same is true for variations in neighbourhood land use and saturated or nonsaturated communities. In the social-status analysis, however, there is some evidence that higher-status neighbourhoods tend to more tolerant of mental health facilities. Such neighbourhoods tend to contain few individuals who would consider moving, and more who would do nothing in response to a facility's opening.

The distance variable measured respondent proximity to a facility in five zones: less than 100 m, 101–200 m, 201–300 m, 301–400 m, and over 500 m. Both the straight-line and block-front distance measures were transformed into these categories, since standard regression tests on the raw distance measures produced no significant results (Boeckh, 1980, page 78). The categorical analysis summarized here proved to be significant in two categories (table 8.6). Consider first the perceived externality impact. For the block-front distance data, significant Kruskal–Wallis statistics were observed for facility impact on personal safety, visual appearance, and undesirable people (all significant at the $0 \cdot 05$ level). For the straight-line distance subsample, similar levels of significance were observed for two variables: personal safety and effect on property values. However, in none of these instances is there a consistent distance-decay relationship in the pattern of observed responses across the various respondent subpopulations.

Finally, there also seems to be a significant, although slight, relationship between distance and behavioural response in some neighbourhoods. However, once again, no clearly discernable, consistent trend is perceptible.

Table 8.6. Summary of statistical tests on disaggregated population samples. (Source: Boeckh, 1980, chapter 5.)

Level of disaggregation (number of categories)	N	Test	Externality impact	Facility desirability by distance	Behavioural response
Social status (3) (two tests)	48 99	K–W	ns	ns	s
Land-use mix (3)	40	K–W	ns	ns	ns
Facility type (2)	49	K–S	ns	ns	ns
Neighbourhood saturation (2)	37	K–S	ns	ns	ns
Distance (5) (two measures)	379	K–W	s	ns	s

ns no significant results in any category. s significant results in some, but not all, categories. K–S Kolmogorov–Smirnov test. K–W Kruskal–Wallis test.

8.6 Discussion
The existence of a range of external effects in association with community mental health facilities has been confirmed. Residents seem to fear the negative effect of such facilities on property values, traffic volumes, and residential satisfaction. However, there is a strongly 'neutral' core of respondents, who essentially believe that such facilities have no impact on

local neighbourhoods. Respondents who claim to be aware of a local mental health facility are relatively more tolerant in their estimation of the neighbourhood impact of mental health facilities, and even appear to anticipate certain positive neighbourhood advantages of a facility's introduction.

The impact of the community mental health facility externality field is spatially very confined. Generally, as proximity to a potential facility increases, so does the perceived undesirability of that facility. The most negative responses tend to occur within one block of a facility location, but beyond a distance of six blocks a more tolerant attitude is evidenced. Both awareness of a facility and type of local facility appear to have some effect on the results, although proximity to the source of the external effects is clearly the dominant factor conditioning respondent perception. The mental health facility appears to be a classic 'noxious facility', in that it is generally regarded as a necessary service, but it is least welcomed by residents closest to a potential site.

Behavioural adjustments in response to the mental health facility's externality field are surprisingly limited. Fully one-third of a subsample (which rated a facility as undesirable) would do nothing in response to a facility's introduction. However, greater proximity to the facility suggested a greater propensity to become involved especially in group-based opposition tactics. Also significant was the increase in the proportion of respondents who considered moving because of the facility. Awareness of a local mental health facility did little to alter the pattern of behavioural response. Only a very small minority reported actually engaging in active opposition to a facility location.

In the light of these findings, perhaps our assumptions about the negative impact of community mental health facilities ought to be revised. The majority of respondents in this sample seem to be relatively favourably disposed toward community mental health care. Even when survey questions invite consideration of the negative impact of community facilities, the majority respond with 'neutral' assessments. These generally benevolent sentiments are confirmed by the very small minority who seem to evidence active opposition behaviour. It seems likely that a vocal opposition minority (usually with extensive media coverage) can often inflate a local difficulty out of all proportion.

The pattern of response in the Toronto survey may be due, at least in part, to biases in survey structure. For instance, only relatively small-scale facilities were considered in the questionnaire, and some facilities were virtually 'invisible' (one centre operated from the basement of a church, for example). In addition, the survey response was concerned primarily with hypothetical locations; we did not obtain the reactions of residents immediately prior to, during, or after the opening of a specific facility. However, in defence, it may be countered that the survey respondents were drawn from within a rigorous stratified random-sample design. Moreover, the level of recent public debate (in Toronto) over the location of group homes has been very high. Yet our sample demonstrates a relatively low level of awareness of neighbourhood facilities. We therefore conclude that the noncombative, nonaware characteristics of our sample population are seemingly typical of the population at large. Externality-induced opposition to community mental health facilities is therefore probably limited to a vociferous minority whose views may not be representative of the wider community.

The most important theoretical issues raised in this empirical analysis concern the relatively subtle impact of small-scale external effects upon the arrangement of urban space. Even though mental health facilities may be noxious, their spatial impact is locally highly confined, and there seems little doubt that they are also endowed with a positive association of social worth or merit. As a consequence, their impact is minor, and they cannot be regarded as a significant catalyst for readjustment of the population surface. It is likely that major readjustments depend upon other dimensions of the externality source, especially scale. Even then, however, the precise nature of the externality field, and the response it may induce, remains indeterminate. As a consequence, we would suggest that a much greater empirical effort is necessary in order to evaluate some of the theoretical claims made for the role of externalities in the structuring of urban space.

Effects of mental health facilities on neighbourhood property values

Neighbourhood opposition to community-based mental health facilities is often founded upon a fear of diminished property values in their vicinity. Such sentiments appear with monotonous regularity in media accounts of conflict over facility siting, in spite of an almost total absence of systematic evidence on this topic. As the move toward community-based mental health continues, this gap in our knowledge makes it increasingly difficult to respond factually to residents' fears. In the meantime, the future of the mental health delivery system is jeopardized, since its continuing effectiveness is contingent upon successful integration into the neighbourhood setting.

The purpose of this chapter is to provide a systematic assessment of the property value effects of a sample of mental health facilities in Toronto. We wish to establish whether or not there is any basis in fact for the common community fears which we encountered in chapter 8. Although our objective is simply stated, the analytical task is formidable. Hence, in what follows, an attempt is first made to clarify the problems in research design for property value analysis. The selection of sample facilities is then discussed, and in the final section of the chapter the analytical findings are described.

9.1 Property value analysis

The introduction of a mental health facility may be regarded either passively as a neutral event, or as something which brings a positive asset into the community. In both circumstances, the facility would not provoke the residents to relocate, property turnover rates would remain unaffected, and prices might be expected to appreciate normally. However, if the facility is viewed negatively, it could provoke an exodus of nearby residents and severely depress the resale price of properties in its vicinity. Hence, movements in property values can be regarded as a reasonable reflection of aggregate neighbourhood response to the introduction of mental health facilities. Two questions should be addressed initially: what is the existing evidence of such property value movements? and what are the research problems associated with property value analysis?

The effect of mental health facilities on property values has not been widely studied. In one of the few published reports, Dear (1977) concludes that although there was some increase in property market activity in the vicinity of twelve Philadelphia mental health facilities, the anticipated decline in sales prices did not materialize. Moreover, the changes which did occur were associated with general market trends rather than with the impact of any specific facility. This early study, however, is flawed because the data were not discounted to take account of inflation.

A similar absence of property effects was noted in a study of seventeen community mental health facilities in White Plains, NY. Although his results were 'inconclusive' because of various data limitations, Breslow (1976, page 18) suggests that communities can absorb a 'limited number' of group homes without measurable effects.

More recently, the market effects associated with group homes for the mentally retarded have been examined. For instance, Wolpert (1978) assessed the impact of forty-two sites within ten cities in New York State. He concluded that markets in the vicinity of the facilities were not significantly different from those in matched control areas (although the control sites were in relatively close proximity to the facility sites). Sale prices did not decline, nor was there a significantly higher degree of property turnover in the vicinity of the facilities. Similarly, in an informal study of group homes for the retarded in Toronto, no significant depreciation was recorded (Metropolitan Toronto Association for the Mentally Retarded, 1979).

In the Ottawa region, Goodale and Wickware (1979) examined the property effect of group homes for ex-prisoners, the mentally retarded, and children. Five indicators were developed: rate of turnover, selling price, annual rates of appreciation, number of days properties were listed before sales, and actual selling price as a percentage of asking price. They found that there was no evidence either of property values or of market-ability being adversely affected by the presence of group homes in residentially zoned neighbourhoods.

These tentative interpretations of property value effects are not solely a reflection of the small number of research studies that have been under-taken. Acute inferential problems are posed by the general class of property value impact analyses. Five problems are particularly relevant:
1. A primary difficulty is associated with the need to define a relevant impact area for analysis. This delimitation must occur before analysis can begin, but there are few a priori criteria to guide definition (Rothenburg, 1967). A too narrowly defined impact area would tend to underestimate the extent of the property value externality field; conversely, a too broadly defined area would risk diluting the property value impact. It is customary, under these circumstances, to resort to rule-of-thumb principles based upon field experience, but some analysis of the stability of the results, using different-sized impact areas, ought also to be undertaken if data sources permit.
2. The problem of controlling for 'noise' in the data analysis is equally troublesome. It is literally impossible to hold all other variables constant while selected impact indicators are being examined. Hence, sale price may be more influenced by property condition than by the introduction of a new facility. Alternatively, some far-distant change in the transportation network may induce an accessibility-related change in market conditions which could obscure the facility's impact. Finally, as Schall (1971) has

indicated, the values of land and structure can often move in different directions, and the net effect will depend upon the relative magnitudes of these two discrete changes. In the face of such complexity, inferential problems are great, and we continue to lack research designs which would permit the role of individual variables to be definitively identified in any given causal sequence.

3. The problem of scale is also pertinent here. When the source of the property effect is large-scale, there is usually little doubt about the cause-and-effect relationship. There is further substantial confirmation if the property effect diminishes with increased distance from the source (Hammer et al, 1971). However, the types of mental health facilities in this study are very small-scale. They are frequently no larger than a common row house (in the case of a group home), a store-front (drop-in centre), or a branch library (an outpatient unit). It is all too easy for their property effects to be submerged by general market conditions.

4. It may be suggested that many of these difficulties would be resolved by judicious selections of a suitable control neighbourhood against which to assess changes in the sample data. However, it is never possible to duplicate exactly the conditions of individual neighbourhood property markets. Similarity in sociodemographic structure is no guarantee that property markets will be alike. It may be possible to select the sample and the control from within one broadly homogeneous neighbourhood, as Wolpert (1978) did, but this puts the independence of the two markets at risk.

5. Last, there is a class of problems which involves some form of discounting for various inconsistencies in the property value data. Because data are almost inevitably collected for nonuniform time periods, and because there is bound to be an irregular volume and spacing of sales transactions in the vicinity of any facility, some method of averaging, or discounting, has to be found (Taylor et al, 1982). For example, Dear (1977) collected data on average value of sales transactions for periods of two years before and after the introduction of a facility. In addition, even over a short time period, a further discounting must be undertaken to offset the effect of inflation.

In summary, a proper research design for property value analysis would require a reasonable a priori definition of the impact area of a facility; a clearly defined causal model which would eliminate exogenous 'noise', and permit reliable inferences about the effect of small-scale facilities, the specification of an adequate control sample, and proper discounting procedures to compensate for variations in the sample frame.

9.2 Analytical approach and sampling procedures

The principles described above were used to develop a three-stage analytical approach. First, the effect of the introduction of a mental health facility on the volume of sales activity was examined. An increase in the number of property transactions could be anticipated immediately prior to, during, or after the opening of a facility. Second, the effect of facility introduction on sale price was tested. A decline in price paid for properties in the vicinity of a facility may be expected as a consequence of a decrease in housing demand. Care was taken to control for the effects of inflation on prices, and to standardize prices on the basis of price per room. Third, the effects on sale price of different facility characteristics were tested using multiple regression analysis. By means of controls for the effects of dwelling unit and neighbourhood variables, the effects of the following facility characteristics were assessed: the presence or absence of a facility, distance from a facility, type of facility, and number of facilities.

To conduct these analyses, real estate and land-use data were collected for areas in the vicinity of five community mental health facilities in Toronto. Four group homes and one outpatient unit were included, all purposely selected from the larger facility set described in chapter 5. The major concern was not that they should be representative of the total set of facilities in the metropolitan area, but that they should be removed from other types of facilities which would be likely to affect the local property market. To this end, the study sample was chosen from areas without major transportation arteries, other public facilities, or any other land uses likely to exert a confounding property value impact.

The baseline data for sales transactions was defined as the month of facility opening. Data on transactions were collected by quarterly periods for the two years before and after the introduction of the facility. Because of ambiguities concerning the opening date of two facilities (numbers 2 and 5), only the year of opening was available. However, data were still assembled for the two years before and after in these special cases.

Table 9.1. Neighbourhood and facility characteristics. (Source: Boeckh et al, 1980, page 277.)

Characteristic	Facility information number				
	1	2	3	4	5
Facility type [a]	GH	GH	OP	GH	GH
Location [b]	C	C	C	S	S
Neighbourhood status [c]	U	M	L	M	L
Neighbourhood land use [d]					
commercial	3·7	0·0	28·3	7·9	3·6
single-family	0·0	0·0	0·0	48·2	22·4
multiple-family	69·3	97·2	66·1	30·8	65·5
Time period [e]	4·74–	1·71–	4·73–	1·73–	1·69–
	2·78	4·75	7·77	4·76	4·73

[a] GH—group home; OP—outpatient; [b] C—city, S—suburb; [c] U—upper class, M—middle class, L—lower class; [d] figures expressed as percentages; [e] time periods for property transactions are divided into quarterly periods for each year (for example, 4·74 refers to the fourth quarter, October–December, of 1974).

For each facility an impact area with a radius of 400 m was defined, and all housing sales (except condominiums and sheriff's sales) within these areas were recorded by use of the 'multiple listing service' records of the Toronto Real Estate Board. In each case, data were collected on the terms of the sale and on a variety of housing characteristics. In addition, the impact area surrounding each facility was divided into four concentric distance zones, each ring with a width of 100 m, so that sales could be coded according to distance from the facility. The land-use mix in each area was also calculated from zoning maps and a field survey (table 9.1). Last, a control area was selected for each facility area according to the same criteria employed in the facility selection, and on the basis of locational and socioeconomic comparability. The same data were then collected for each control area for time periods identical to the paired facility area. A sample of 1261 sales was assembled, composed of 560 within the facility areas and 701 in the control areas.

Using these procedures, we hoped to define an operational research design for property value analysis. Needless to say, our design did not totally match the stringent requirements established in the preceding section. In particular, it must be immediately apparent that the 400 m impact area definition is arbitrary. We anticipated that the division into 100 m zones would allow for a systematic test of varying the geographical extent of the property effect. However, in many instances, the number of sales within each zone was too small to enable any such analysis. On all other counts, we believe that the research design outlined here is adequate for the task.

9.3 The property value effect
9.3.1 Sales activity
The effect of a facility on sales activity was examined by comparing the number of property transactions in the facility and matched control areas. The comparison was made for three time periods: before, during, and after the introduction of the facility (table 9.2). The actual percentage of sales in each area was compared with the expected percentage of sales expressed as the percentage of the total survey period in each time period (table 9.3).

Consider first the aggregate percentages for the facility and control areas. These generally correspond quite closely with the expected percentages. For the first two time periods, the percentages for the facility areas are higher than for the control areas. For period 3 the opposite applies. This reversal is certainly inconsistent with the hypothesis that the introduction of a facility causes an increase in sales activity.

Larger differences between actual and expected percentages are observed when the individual facility areas are examined. However, the direction of the differences is inconsistent. For the third and probably most crucial time period, the actual exceeds the expected percentage of sales for areas

Table 9.2. Number of transactions by time period. (Source: Boeckh et al, 1980, page 277.)

Area	Period 1[a]	Period 2[b]	Period 3[c]	Total
1	23	4	26	53
Control	66	8	52	126
2	49	29	46	124
Control	63	23	82	168
3	106	19	68	193
Control	125	11	116	252
4	46	9	64	119
Control	23	3	49	75
5	23	20	28	71
Control	23	20	37	80
All facility areas	247	81	232	560
All control areas	300	65	336	701

[a] Period 1: two years prior to facility introduction (twenty-one months only for facilities 4 and 5 because of data unavailability). [b] Period 2: period of facility introduction (one quarter for facilities 1, 3, and 4; one year for facilities 2 and 5). [c] Period 3: two years following facility introduction (eighteen months only for facility 1—data available to mid-1978 only).

Table 9.3. Percentage of total sales compared with percentage of total survey time by period[a]. (Source: Boeckh et al, 1980, page 278.)

Area	Period 1		Period 2		Period 3	
	% sales	% time	% sales	% time	% sales	% time
1	43·4	53·3	7·6	6·7	49·1	40·0
Control	52·4	53·3	6·4	6·7	41·3	40·0
2	39·5	40·0	23·4	20·0	37·1	40·0
Control	37·5	40·0	13·7	20·0	48·8	40·0
3	54·9	47·1	9·9	5·9	35·2	47·1
Control	49·6	47·1	4·4	5·9	46·0	47·1
4	38·7	43·8	7·6	6·3	53·8	50·0
Control	30·7	43·8	4·0	6·3	65·3	50·1
5	32·5	36·9	28·2	21·1	39·4	42·1
Control	28·8	36·9	25·0	21·1	46·3	42·1
All facility areas	44·1	43·7	14·5	12·7	41·4	43·7
All control areas	42·8	43·7	9·3	12·7	48·0	43·7
Total sample	43·4	43·7	11·6	12·7	45·0	43·7

[a] Percentage of total sales (% sales) and percentage of total survey time (% time) are given by

$$\% \text{ sales} = \frac{\text{number of sales for period } j \text{ in area } i}{\text{total sales in area } i} \times 100$$

$$\% \text{ time} = \frac{\text{number of months in period } j \text{ for area } i}{\text{total number of months surveyed for area } i} \times 100$$

1 and 4, and falls below it for the other three areas. Comparing the actual percentages for each facility–control pair for time period 3 reveals some further inconsistency. In the case of the first pair, the percentage is higher for the facility area; but in the other four pairs, the percentage is higher for the control area. The evidence again shows no increase in sales activity following facility introduction. It is also important to notice that the data provide no clear evidence of a *reduction* in sales activity in facility areas, as might be predicted if the new facility caused a decline in housing demand.

9.3.2 Sale price

The lack of an effect on sales *activity* does not exclude the possibility that the introduction of a facility may affect sale *price*. Sale prices were examined by comparing the average prices of housing transactions in each facility and control area for each of the three time periods.

In absolute terms, after facility introduction, average house prices rose 20·9% for the facility areas compared with an increase of only 12·4% for the control areas. However, caution is necessary in interpreting absolute figures, because the differences in average sale price may reflect differences in housing characteristics as well as differences in inflation rates. To control for inflation effects, individual house prices were deflated to 1969 (first quarter) values. Deflation factors were calculated for each of three Toronto submarkets (east, west, and central Toronto) for quarterly time

Table 9.4. Deflated mean sale price per room in 10^3 Can $ by period and by percentage changes from period 1 to period 2 and from period 2 to period 3. (Source: Boeckh et al, 1980, page 280.)

Area	Period 1		Period 2		Period 3		Change (%)	
	MSP	SD	MSP	SD	MSP	SD	1–2	2–3
1	3·38	1·04	3·28	1·25	3·46	0·88	−2·96	5·49
Control	4·33	0·86	4·51	0·82	4·25	0·84	4·16	5·76
2	3·61	0·76	3·29	0·66	3·33	0·79	−8·86	1·22
3	2·38	0·67	2·69	0·71	2·81	0·80	1·53	8·54
Control	2·41	0·51	2·70	0·60	2·91	0·71	12·03	7·78
4	2·33	1·25	2·64	0·91	2·90	0·78	13·30	9·85
Control	3·37	0·72	3·98	0·94	4·37	0·75	18·10	9·80
5	1·76	1·55	1·74	0·82	2·06	0·88	−1·14	18·39
Control	2·17	1·50	1·89	0·73	3·66	0·75	5·25	7·33
All facility areas	2·69	1·05	2·73	0·82	2·91	0·83	1·49	6·59
All control areas	3·24	0·76	3·41	0·73	3·66	0·75	5·25	7·33
Total	2·97	0·91	3·07	0·77	3·29	0·79	3·37	7·17

[a] All values deflated to 1969 (first quarter) values.
MSP deflated mean sale price; SD standard deviation.

periods, by use of data on monthly average sale prices obtained from the
Toronto Real Estate Board (Toronto Real Estate Board, 1978). In this
way, spatial variations in house price changes were incorporated to reflect
differences in inflation rates between housing submarkets. Second, to
control for major variations in housing characterisitcs the deflated house
price was converted to price per room. These deflated standardized figures
were then used to calculate the average sale price per room for each
facility and control area (table 9.4).

Average sale price per room in the facility areas shows an increase of
1·5% between periods 1 and 2, and 6·6% between periods 2 and 3. The
corresponding figures for the control areas are 5·3% and 7·3%. The
increases in sale price in the facility areas both prior to and following
facility introduction, and the higher rate of increase between periods 2 and
3, are further indications that the opening of facilities has not caused a
drop in sale prices. However, the percentage increases are lower in the
facility than in the control areas, but the differences are small. Comparison
with sale prices in the control areas suggests that prices in the facility areas
have generally increased at a comparable rate.

9.3.3 Effects of facility characteristics on property values
The possible effect of neighbourhood mental health facilities on residential
property values was further examined by a series of regression analyses.
The dependent variable for each analysis was the sale price for period 3
(the two-year period following facility introduction), deflated to 1969
(first quarter) prices. The independent variables of primary interest were
those related to variation in facility characteristics, but to assess the
influence of these variables on sale price, it was essential to include other
variables in the regression equations to control for common features known
to influence house prices. Three sets of control factors were included:
housing variables (lot size, number of rooms, number of garage spaces, and
number of bathrooms), a dummy location variable (city or suburb), and a
land-use variable (percentage of neighbourhood devoted to commercial land
use).

The regression analyses are important in that they introduce both a
greater inferential precision into the analysis, as well as a consideration of
several facility characteristics which could influence neighbourhood
property markets. The four regression analyses, and their variables, were
as follows:
1. the presence or absence of a facility in a neighbourhood (the simplest
of initial causal models);
2. the distance of transacted properties from the local facility (an acutely
important test, because without a consistent distance-decay effect, any
property market perturbation cannot logically be ascribed to the facility
source);

3. the type of facility (since resident perceptions are likely to be sensitive to differences in facility design, operating characteristics, etc); and
4. number of facilities (the 'saturation' dimension, and its potential effect on property sales).
Separate regression tests, using different subsets of the sample data, were performed to determine the role of each of these four characteristics. In all cases, sale price was used as the dependent variable.

The first analysis was designed to assess the effect of the presence of a facility in a neighbourhood and used the data for all ten control and facility areas. The presence or absence of a facility was included in the equation as a dummy variable (0—no facility, 1—facility). The results (table 9.5) indicate that all six independent variables were significant, and together accounted for 70% of the variation in sale price, with the number of rooms being by far the most powerful predictor.

The presence of a facility was significant, although it accounted for only $1 \cdot 3\%$ of the explained variation in sale price. The regression coefficient $(-2 \cdot 358)$ shows that, with controls for the other five independent variables in the equation, sale price in areas with facilities were on average Can $2358 lower than in the control areas. We tentatively conclude therefore that the presence of a facility has a weak effect on property values.

The second analysis examines whether this weak effect varies systematically with the distance within facility areas. Distance was measured in terms of four 100 m zones around the facility location. All seven independent variables satisfied conditions for entry into the equation (table 9.6), but the distance variable was the only one that was not significant. As the last variable included in the stepwise procedure, it accounted for only a $0 \cdot 1\%$ increase in the explained variation in sale price. The remaining six variables in the equation together accounted for 85% of the variance, with number of rooms again being by far the most powerful predictor. The absence of a consistent distance-decay effect in the pattern of sale price variation may be due partly to the arbitrary definition of the impact area (a 400 m radius from a facility). However, its much more

Table 9.5. Multiple regression analysis testing the effect of facility presence on sale price ($N = 568$)[a]. (Source: Boeckh et al, 1980, page 281.)

Variable	B	β	R^2	Change in R^2
Number of rooms	$1 \cdot 180$	$0 \cdot 373$	$0 \cdot 534$	$0 \cdot 534$
Number of bathrooms	$2 \cdot 015$	$0 \cdot 273$	$0 \cdot 570$	$0 \cdot 036$
Lot size	$0 \cdot 002$	$0 \cdot 367$	$0 \cdot 604$	$0 \cdot 034$
Location dummy	$7 \cdot 193$	$0 \cdot 307$	$0 \cdot 677$	$0 \cdot 073$
Facility dummy	$-2 \cdot 358$	$-0 \cdot 107$	$0 \cdot 690$	$0 \cdot 013$
Number of garages	$1 \cdot 145$	$0 \cdot 093$	$0 \cdot 696$	$0 \cdot 006$
Constant	ns			

[a] All values significant at the $0 \cdot 001$ level; ns not significant.

important implication is that the property effect shown in the preceding
equation (table 9.5) is not necessarily due to the presence of a facility,
but may be more properly associated with other extraneous market factors.

The third regression tested the effect of facility type on sale price.
Sales data were assembled for a neighbourhood with an outpatient unit
(facility 3) and a neighbourhood with a group home (facility 5). Type
of facility was included in the analysis as a dummy variable (0—outpatient
unit; 1—group home), but it made no significant contribution to the
equation. In fact it failed to meet the requirement of the stepwise
procedure for entry into the computation. The four significant independent
variables—number of rooms, percentage of commercial land use, lot size,
and number of bathrooms—together accounted for 63% of the variation
in sale price (table 9.7). From these results, it is evident that facility type
has no significant effect on sale price.

Finally, the effect of the number of facilities in a neighbourhood was
examined. Sales data in this case were drawn from two neighbourhoods,
one with four group homes (facility A), and a second with only one group
home (facility B). Number of facilities was therefore dichotomous and

Table 9.6. Multiple regression analysis testing the effect of distance from facility on
sale price ($N = 232$)[a]. (Source: Boeckh et al, 1980, page 282.)

Variable	B	β	R^2	Change in R^2
Number of rooms	1·123	0·357	0·739	0·739
Number of bathrooms	2·198	0·312	0·768	0·029
Location dummy	9·824	0·328	0·794	0·026
Lot size	0·001	0·180	0·828	0·034
% Commercial land use	−0·161	−0·124	0·842	0·014
Number of garages	1·847	0·131	0·852	0·010
Distance	ns	0·036	0·853	0·001
Constant	ns			

[a] All values significant at the 0·001 level; ns not significant.

Table 9.7. Multiple regression analysis testing the effect of facility type on sale price
($N = 96$)[a]. (Source: Boeckh et al, 1980, page 282.)

Variable	B	β	R^2	Change in R^2
Number of rooms	0·924	0·325	0·299	0·299
% Commercial land use	0·495	0·823	0·488	0·189
Lot size	0·002	0·504	0·613	0·125
Number of bathrooms	ns	0·135	0·630	0·017
Number of garages	ns	0·075	0·634	0·004
Constant	−7·670			

[a] All values significant at the 0·001 level; ns not significant.

was defined as a dummy variable (0—more than one facility; 1—one facility). As in the previous analysis, the facility saturation variable failed to meet the requirements for entry into the regression equation (table 9.8), which suggests that the number of facilities in a neighbourhood had no significant effect on sale price. The five significant control variables in this analysis were number of rooms, lot size, number of bathrooms, percentage of commercial land use, and number of garage spaces. These variables in combination, accounted for 91% of the variation in sale price.

Taken together, the four regression analyses show that in only one instance did the location of mental health facilities have a significant effect on house prices. Sales prices in neighbourhoods with existing facilities were, on average, Can \$2358 lower than in control areas without facilities. However, the lack of a systematic distance-decay effect in the pattern of sales price suggests that this price differential cannot be conclusively linked to the presence of a facility. For those areas with facilities, neither type of facility nor number of facilities had any measurable effect on sale price.

Table 9.8. Multiple regression analysis testing the effect of number of facilities on sale price ($N = 72$)[a]. (Source: Boeckh et al, 1980, page 283.)

Variable	B	β	R^2	Change in R^2
Number of rooms	0·961	0·326	0·851	0·851
Lot size	0·003	0·235	0·871	0·020
Number of bathrooms	2·003	0·324	0·893	0·022
% Commercial land use	1·496	0·129	0·907	0·014
Number of garages	1·585	0·112	0·912	0·005
Constant	5·733			

[a] All values significant at the 0·05 level.

9.4 Summary

This chapter has examined the effect of a sample of mental health facilities upon local property values. There was no evidence that the volume of sales activity was either greater or less in facility than in control areas before, during, or after facility introduction. It could not be concluded that the property market in the facility areas had 'bottomed out' because of lack of demand, as there was no evidence of decline in sale prices in these areas. In facility areas, house prices tended to increase at a comparable rate to those in the control areas. The most important factors influencing house prices were the typical features of the housing units themselves, particularly the number of rooms. Other neighbourhood-related characteristics (city or suburban location, land-use mix) had only a minor effect upon property values. Although the presence of a facility was associated with a small reduction in property values, doubts about the causality of this association remain because none of the other three facility characteristics (distance, type, number) emerged as significant variables in the regression tests.

We conclude that property market movements in our sample of Toronto neighbourhoods are due mainly to such traditional factors as neighbourhood desirability and characteristics of the housing unit being sold. The introduction of a mental health facility has no conclusive effect on neighbourhood property values.

10   Profiles of accepting and rejecting neighbourhoods

This chapter considers the problems of planning for the location of mental health facilities. The extensive task of planning facility locations requires a relatively simple, easily applied method for anticipating neighbourhood response to proposed facility sites. A survey such as ours is simply impractical for every siting decision. Hence, the need (in planning terms) is for a simple research tool which employs easily available data and which provides a good estimate of aggregate social response on a neighbourhood basis. The purpose of this chapter is to outline one possible methodology for profiling those communities which are likely either to accept or reject a neighbourhood mental health facility.

10.1 The planning problem
In a nutshell, planning for social services may be described as an exercise in matching client needs to a range of appropriate treatment settings[4]. Client needs range from those in need of total life support to those who need only incidental support in their everyday life patterns. This distinction recognizes the polar extremes of need, between complete client *dependence* (for example, profound retardation) to relative client *autonomy* (for example, occasional counselling), and suggests a full range of gradations between the two poles. To meet these needs, an equivalent taxonomy of treatment settings is implied. At the one end of the spectrum is the *closed protected* environment (an asylum); at the other end, the *open unrestricted* environment (a drop-in centre), with a range of treatment environments between them. The task of service delivery involves assessing client needs and then assigning the client to the appropriate treatment setting. The objective in assignment is twofold: to minimize the discrepancy between the actual and the preferred assignment, and to minimize the degree of client 'envelopment' in the service system. It is easy to see how mismatches can arise in the delivery of care. For instance, it is often very difficult to to provide an accurate assessment of a client's problems and needs; alternatively, underprovision in the service network might lead to gaps in the hierarchy of treatment settings, and clients might be mismatched by this defect on the supply side.

The technical problem of client assessment and assignment is further complicated by the politics of service delivery (compare section 2.1.2). The actual service outcome (for example, the provision or nonprovision of care) is a function of the impact of four principal 'actors' in the planning 'game'. These are the professional care-providers, the city planners, the

---

[4] The following description relies heavily on the model developed by Dear and Wolch (1980).

clients in need, and the host community. Each of these groups brings their own objectives, skills, and resources to bear on the service problem. Thus, the actual pattern of service delivery will depend upon how these groups converge and impinge upon each other in the service decision. The precise dynamics of this interaction are outside the scope of this chapter (compare Greenblat, 1978). Instead, we focus only on our direct concern in this book—the community.

The community plays a vital role in the success or failure of a neighbourhood-based mental health care system (see, for example, the reports submitted to the President's Commission on Mental Health, 1978). An accepting host community can facilitate the resocialization of the ex-psychiatric patient; a rejecting community is likely only to aggravate the already profound difficulties of reintegration. In one of the few studies in the dynamics of community integration of the mentally ill, Segal and Aviram (1978) identified three groups of factors influencing the integration process: (a) community characteristics, including facility location and proximity to community resources, (b) characteristics of facility residents, and (c) the characteristics of the facility itself. (The construct is certainly supported by the findings in this study.) In a related analysis, Trute and Segal (1976) tried to identify supportive communities for the severely mentally disabled. Such communities appeared to be those in which there exists neither strong cohesion nor severe social dislocation. The former tends to 'close ranks' against the client; the latter tends to be too chaotic and threatening. A number of studies by C J Smith emphasize the importance of client motivation and of the host environment in determining a client's ability to remain out of hospital. Personal characteristics influencing the recidivism rate include the extent of the desire to leave hospital, current hospital experience, family and living situation, aftercare arrangements, and employment (Smith and Smith, 1978). Once discharged, the quality of the outside environment becomes critical for the client's success. According to Smith (1976b), a 'humane' environment is determined by the commercial/industrial character of the setting, housing density, and population transience.

In summary, it seems evident that there is an increasing consensus amongst researchers on the role of the community in the success or failure of neighbourhood-based mental health care. In the following section we attempt to derive a simple parsimonious method for assessing community response.

10.2 A methodology for predicting neighbourhood acceptance or rejection
A fundamental problem of immediate relevance is this: What exactly constitutes acceptance or rejection of a mental health facility? Acceptance could be measured anywhere between community involvement in the facility's activities and the absence of community opposition. Conversely, rejection could involve violent physical assault on a centre and its users or

the signing of a petition. The structure of our questionnaire places limits
on the extent to which this issue may be pursued. The best measure of
acceptance or rejection in the questionnaire is obtained by the following
question (11):

"How do you rate the desirability of having a community-based mental
health facility located within the following distances of your home?
(a) Seven to twelve blocks, (b) two to six blocks, (c) within one block."

Desirability was measured on a nine-point numeric scale ranging from
extremely desirable to extremely undesirable. Two measures of rejection
were calculated from responses to this question for each of the twenty-one
census tracts represented in the sample of neighbourhoods with existing
mental health facilities. The first measure of rejection is the percentage of
responses to any degree undesirable for each census tract (that is, the sum
of slightly undesirable, moderately undesirable, considerably undesirable,
and extremely undesirable responses as a percentage of all responses).
Second, to examine further the notion that there exists a core of opposition
to any given facility, another measure of rejection was computed, namely
the percentage of the sample population in each census tract rating a
facility as considerably or extremely undesirable. For ease of reference,
these two measures are abbreviated to a very undesirable rating (VU) and
an undesirable rating (U). Both measures were calculated for each of the
three distance zones (table 10.1). It is evident that our sample neighbourhoods are representative of a wide range of opinion, including strong
opposition (for example, tract 314) and support (tract 92). In general
terms, the pattern of distance decay in attitudinal change reflects the
patterns observed in the wider population (see chapter 8). Opposition
tends to increase with greater proximity to a facility.

A third measure of rejection was also considered. This was the percentage
of the tract population opposed to the facility in their neighbourhood
[question 15 (a)]. However, this figure was zero for the majority of sample
census tracts because so few respondents were aware of a facility in their
neighbourhood. This variable is therefore likely to be of limited use for
analytical purposes (table 10.1).

Using these measures of rejection as the dependent variable, we sought
to devise a parsimonious description of neighbourhood social structure
using readily available data which were exogenous to our survey source.
In keeping with previous logic regarding the importance of the physical and
social context for a facility, we selected indicators of land-use structure
and social structure. Land use was determined by analysis of land-use
maps for 1976, updated by field survey, for a radius of 400 m from a
facility site. The set of facilities indicates a representative range of
neighbourhoods—predominantly single-family or multiple-family, or strongly
commercial in character (table 10.2). Social structure was defined by
means of census data. A wide set of possible indicators was initially
correlated with our rejection measures, and a reduced set of twelve

independent variables was chosen. The reduced set was broadly descriptive of population age, education, mobility, ethnicity, marital status, home-ownership, and employment status (table 10.3). These data were assembled for the 1976 and 1971 censuses, to provide some indication of growth and change in our sample neighbourhoods.

Before analysing the results of our tests, one cautionary note is necessary. Our analytical design has incorporated three geographical areas which are not spatially coincident. Specifically, land-use data are collected for a radius of 400 m from a facility, census data are collected on a census tract basis, and our attitudinal data were sampled on an enumeration area basis. As a consequence, the dependent variable acceptance/rejection responses are being 'explained' by reference to two sets of variables descriptive of much larger geographical frames of reference. We have no way of systematically estimating the effect of these differences in scale on the results.

Table 10.1. Measures of 'rejection' in sample neighbourhoods (where figures in each category are percentages of tract respondents, and VU and U mean very undesirable and undesirable, respectively).

Census tract number	Distance from facility in blocks						Opposed to local facility
	7–12		2–6		<1		
	VU	U	VU	U	VU	U	
4	0	4·2	4·2	8·4	12·5	12·5	8·3
7	0	0·7	7·1	14·2	14·3	21·4	14·3
18	11·1	11·1	11·1	22·2	33·3	33·3	0
21	0	20·0	10·0	25·0	20·0	30·0	0
32	11·1	11·1	22·2	22·2	33·3	44·4	11·1
91	0	0	0	5·3	10·5	36·8	5·3
91B	0	5·3	10·5	21·0	21·1	36·9	15·8
92	0	10·0	0	10·0	10·0	15·0	5·0
101	8·3	8·3	16·6	24·9	25·0	41·7	0
103	10·0	20·0	20·0	40·0	30·0	30·0	0
116	0	23·5	23·5	23·5	29·4	35·3	11·8
131	4·5	22·7	18·2	31·8	36·4	40·9	0
131B	0	4·8	9·5	19·1	28·6	38·2	0
202	0	20·0	10·0	30·0	30·0	30·0	20·0
208	0	12·5	12·5	21·8	20·9	37·6	0
212	0	0	0	8·3	16·6	24·9	0
219	0	10·0	15·0	25·0	25·0	50·0	0
312	0	15·8	20·3	47·4	31·6	52·7	0
314	0	42·9	14·3	85·8	71·5	85·8	0
351	3·8	11·5	7·3	19·1	15·3	30·6	0
353	8·1	10·1	10·2	26·5	28·6	45·0	0
Sample mean	3·2	11·8	24·0	10·1	38·3	24·6	1·7

Table 10.2. Land use within 400 m of facility (acreages).

Census tract	Land use			
	open space (public)	single-family	multiple-family	commercial[a]
004	8·8	0	70·5	19·9
007	0	0	62·2	37·9
018	4·1	0	50·4	45·6
021	5·6	0	66·1	28·3
032	2·1	0	72·9	25·0
091	0·6	0	70·8	28·9
092	1·3	0	79·7	8·7
101	2·1	0	87·5	10·4
103	2·8	0	97·2	0
116	3·3	31·4	56·9	8·4
131	12·5	58·7	18·3	4·3
202	3·9	48·2	30·8	17·1
208	0·7	14·8	10·9	73·6
212	0	22·4	65·5	12·2
219	0·7	88·3	0	11·0
312	0	42·9	52·1	2·8
314	4·9	0	29·8	65·3
315	4·9	0	29·8	65·3
351	6·1	62·0	21·1	10·8
353	21·1	74·2	0	4·7

[a] Commercial, industrial, and institutional.

Table 10.3. Census variables used as measure of social structure (1971 and 1976)[a].

Population under fifteen years of age
Population over sixty-five years of age
Population with less than grade 9 education
Migrant population (into tract since previous census)
Population with English mother tongue
Single-person households

Population over fifteen years of age and never married
Owner-occupied households
Unemployment rate
Median income[b]
Total population
Population density

[a] Variables measured as percentage of total census tract population.
[b] Available for 1971 census only.

Table 10.4. Regression analysis of neighbourhood profiles.

Independent variable [a]	Dependent variable [a]						
	7–12 blocks		2–6 blocks		<1 block		opposed
	U	VU	U	VU	U	VU	
Equations based on 1976 census data							
Population under 15 years of age	0·51 ns	−0·18 ns	2·43	−0·54 ns	1·80	2·14	−0·36 ns
Population English-speaking	−1·10 **	−[b]	−1·74 *	−0·53 **	−1·10 **	−1·20 **	–
Population homeowners	−0·28 ns	–	–	−0·30 ***	–	0·34 ns	–
Population single-person households	0·22 ns	–	1·03 ***	0·06 ns	0·96 **	1·39 ***	–
Migrant population	−1·07 ***	–	−1·10 ns	−0·62 **	–	−0·83 ns	–
Population with less than grade 9 education	−0·89 ***	0·40 *	−1·67 **	0·36 ns	−0·47 ns	−0·94 ns	–
Population change 1971–1976	–	–	–	0·002	–	–	–
Population density 1976	−0·0005 ns	−0·0002 ***	−0·0008 ns	−0·0006 *	−0·001 **	−0·0005 ns	−0·002 ns
Open space land use	0·46 ns	0·65 *	–	0·61 *	–	0·70 ns	–
Single-family neighbourhood	–	–	–	–	0·17 ns	–	–
Multiple-family neighbourhood	–	0·08 **	–	–	–	–	–
Commercial land use	0·31 ***	–	0·36 ns	–	–	0·41 *	–
Constant	128·09 **	−4·92 ns	138·42 **	86·12 **	93·68 **	54·75 ns	7·01 ns
Adjusted R^2	0·45	0·57	0·59	0·71	0·59	0·53	0·30
Standard error	7·17	2·79	11·03	4·04	9·78	9·08	5·43
Equations based on 1971 to 1976 census data changes							
Population under 15 years of age	−1·16 ns	0·50 ns	−1·54 ns	–	–	–	−1·89 ***
Population homeowners	−1·00 ns	–	−1·59 ns	–	−1·79 ***	–	0·32 ns
Population single-person households	–	−0·47 ns	–	−1·37 ***	−4·42 **	–	–
Migrant population	−0·30 ns	–	0·75 ns	–	0·58 ns	0·54 ns	−0·34 ns
Population with less than grade 9 education	–	–	0·11 ns	0·44 ns	1·35 ns	−0·89 ns	0·29 ns

Population unemployed	–	–	–	–	–	–	–
Population change 1971–1976	–	–	$0 \cdot 003^{ns}$	$0 \cdot 002^{**}$	$0 \cdot 004^{***}$	–	–
Population density 1976	–	$-0 \cdot 002^{ns}$	–	–	$-0 \cdot 003^{ns}$	–	$0 \cdot 004^{ns}$
Open space land use	–	$0 \cdot 37^{***}$	–	–	$-1 \cdot 14^{ns}$	–	–
Single-family neighbourhood	–	$-0 \cdot 01^{ns}$	–	–	$-1 \cdot 67^{**}$	–	–
Multiple-family neighbourhood	–	$0 \cdot 07^{ns}$	–	–	$-1 \cdot 69^{**}$	–	–
Commercial land use	–	–	–	–	$-1 \cdot 37^{***}$	–	–
Constant	$12 \cdot 05^{ns}$	$5 \cdot 05^{ns}$	$36 \cdot 47^{ns}$	$27 \cdot 82^{**}$	$245 \cdot 33^{*}$	$11 \cdot 84^{ns}$	$-5 \cdot 82^{ns}$
Adjusted R^2	$0 \cdot 35$	$0 \cdot 54$	$0 \cdot 38$	$0 \cdot 37$	$0 \cdot 68$	$0 \cdot 27$	$0 \cdot 50$
Standard error	$7 \cdot 84$	$2 \cdot 87$	$13 \cdot 53$	$5 \cdot 96$	$8 \cdot 58$	$11 \cdot 29$	$5 \cdot 02$

[a] All variables expressed as percentages except for population change and population density.
[b] Did not enter computation.
* Significant at the $0 \cdot 001$ level; ** significant at the $0 \cdot 01$ level; *** significant at the $0 \cdot 05$ level; ns not significant at the $0 \cdot 05$ level.

10.2.1 Analysis and results

The analysis involved calculating regression equations to predict the percentage of a population rejecting neighbourhood mental health facilities. Seven rejection measures were used as dependent variables: percentage rejecting, and percentage strongly rejecting, for each of the three facility distances (that is, seven to twelve blocks, two to six blocks, less than one block); and percentage opposed to an existing facility. Two sets of independent variables were used. The first included six 1976 census variables as social indicators (percentage under fifteen years of age, percentage English-speaking, percentage homeowners, percentage single-person households, percentage migrants, percentage with less than grade 9 education). The second included six measures of social change based on the difference between the 1976 and 1971 census data for five of the same six variables, together with percentage unemployed in place of percentage English-speaking. Two other census variables (population change 1971–1976 and 1976 population density) were included in both sets as were four land-use variables: percentage open space, percentage single-family housing, percentage multiple-family housing, and percentage commercial. Given seven rejection measures and two sets of independent variables, a total of fourteen equations were calculated.

A stepwise regression procedure was followed, and the equations maximizing the adjusted R^2 value are reported (table 10.4). (The adjusted R^2 value is a conservative estimate of the explained variation appropriate where the number of cases is small relative to the number of independent variables.) Each equation is significant overall beyond the 95% confidence level. The adjusted R^2 values ranged from $0 \cdot 27$ to $0 \cdot 71$ representing a low to moderate level of explanation allowing for the small number of cases. For most equations there are several independent variables which fail to enter and others which, though entered, make a nonsignificant contribution to the final equation. The initial impression is that neither set of independent variables (the 1976 data nor the 1971–1976 change data) provides a very powerful basis for profiling rejection and accepting communities.

Considered in more detail, the equations based on the 1976 census variables are (with two exceptions) more powerful than the corresponding equations including the 1971–1976 social change measures. It is reasonable therefore to concentrate on the first set of variables in attempting to construct community profiles, especially as they are more easily interpreted. Inspection of the regression coefficients reveals a number of variables which behave consistently in two or more equations (that is, they are statistically significant in the same direction). This consistency is evident for percentage population under fifteen years of age and percentage of single-person households census variables; and for percentage of open space and percentage commercial land-use variables. Rejection increases with increasing scores on each of these four variables. In contrast, rejection decreases with percentage English-speaking population, percentage migrant population, and population density census variables. The coefficients for two equations also indicate increasing rejection in relation to percentage population with less than grade 9 education. A third equation (for percentage population with a strong rejection at a distance of seven to twelve blocks) shows the opposite relationship, but this particular equation is suspect because the majority of scores on the dependent variable are zero (table 10.1) and hence the parameters are strongly affected by responses in a very small number of census tracts.

There is less consistency in the pattern of regression coefficients for the equations based on the 1971 to 1976 changes in census data. There is limited evidence that rejection is higher in areas which have experienced the greatest growth in population over the five-year period. Equally, there are indications of lower levels of rejection in areas which have experienced increases in the proportion of homeowners and single-person households. Neither of these last two relationships is easily interpreted, and both are somewhat counterintuitive.

10.2.2 Discussion

The immediate question is whether these results provide a reliable basis for profiling the characteristics of accepting and rejecting neighbourhoods. The subsequent question is whether the profile characteristics observed from these data correspond with those suggested by previous studies, and further whether they correspond with the correlates of individual attitudes toward the mentally ill and mental health facilities reported in earlier chapters.

The initial answer to the first question is that no strong profile either of accepting or of rejecting neighbourhoods emerges. This conclusion is based both on the limited explanatory power of the regression equations and on the lack of significance in the contributions of the specific independent variables. Nevertheless, there are, as previously described, some consistencies in the pattern of relationships which are a basis for identifying preliminary profiles. In this respect the results based on the 1976 census variables are the most useful. From those results we tentatively conclude that *accepting* neighbourhoods are those in which residents have few children, are well-educated, and predominantly English speaking; where the population is relatively transient, the population density relatively high; and where there is a mixture of land uses with commercial development and public open space in addition to residential areas. It follows, therefore, that *rejecting* neighbourhoods tend to be those in which there are younger children, low education levels, and non-English-speaking groups represented; where the population has been relatively stable over the past five years and population density is low; and where the land use is predominantly residential (table 10.5).

To what extent to these profiles correspond to those suggested in previous studies? The limited available evidence (for example, Armstrong, 1976; Trute and Segal, 1976) seems to correspond quite closely. As discussed in chapter 2, acceptance is higher in areas of mixed land use and low levels of social cohesion, as characterized by a low proportion of married couples and by correspondingly high rates of single-person households. On the other hand, rejection has been shown to be higher in highly cohesive neighbourhoods, typically in suburban areas with a predominance of nuclear families and homogeneity in terms of race, class, and educational background. Although there is not a total correspondence between these earlier findings and the present results, the overlap is considerable and adds credibility to our findings.

There is also a reasonable degree of correspondence between these results and those reported in chapter 7 (based on the individual-level data). There it was shown that community mental health orientation is stronger for those who are young, female, single, without children, are well-educated, and who rent their homes. The overlap with the results from the aggregate data described in this chapter is clear, although again there is not complete correspondence. (The absence of a significant effect for homeownership in the aggregate data is one notable example.) The ecological fallacy warns us against expecting correspondence between the results based on different units of analysis. Nevertheless, finding it to the extent evident here is reassuring in terms of the reliability of the aggregate results.

Table 10.5. Profiles of accepting and rejecting neighbourhoods.

Accepting neighbourhoods	Rejecting neighbourhoods
Few children	Many children
Well-educated	Lower education levels
English-speaking	Non-English-speaking groups
Transient population	Stable population
High population density	Low population density
Mixed land use	Predominantly residential

10.3 Geographical distribution of existing mental health facilities in Toronto

An obvious question is to what extent does the geographical distribution of *existing* mental health facilities in Toronto match the *predicted* distribution implied by the results of the previous section? We must approach this question with caution, because the presence or absence of a strong association between existing and predicted distributions can be only partly explained by our analytical focus, that is, community attitudes.

Other factors which have demonstrably influenced the existing facility distribution are:
conflict-minimizing strategies of planners,
facility architecture and design,
availability of large properties suitable for conversion to community
    mental health centres,
conflict over siting decisions (associated with exclusionary or non-
    exclusionary accepting behaviour of residents),
professional practices of assignment and referral,
planning strategies (especially those seeking to minimize conflict), and
spatial distribution of potential users and their needs.

A systematic analysis of the dynamics of facility siting decisions, taking into account all these variables, is beyond the scope of this book. However, it will be of interest briefly to compare predicted and existing distributions as an exploratory step in initiating the next phases of the research undertaken here.

10.3.1 Neighbourhood characteristics and the existing pattern of facility distribution [5]

The geographical distribution of Toronto mental health facilities is clearly very localized. Many suburban boroughs in Metropolitan Toronto are almost totally devoid of any facilities, whereas the inner core of the City of Toronto houses ghetto-like concentrations of facilities (for example, Parkdale, to the southwest of the central area; see figure 10.1). To determine the socioeconomic correlates of the existing distribution of facilities, three analytical problems had to be overcome; (1) the geographical scale of analysis, (2) the measure of facility concentration, and (3) the selection of socioeconomic indicators.

For analytical purposes, two geographic units were selected: (a) census tract and (b) planning district. Each individual tract comprises between 2500 and 8000 people, with lower numbers in the central city. Tract size ranges from $8 \cdot 10$ to $54 \cdot 21$ km^2, with a general increase in size with distance from the city centre (figure 10.1). Two types of planning districts are relevant: those for which we possess survey and socioeconomic data, and those for which we possess only socioeconomic data (figure 10.2).

Facility concentration was defined for each tract and planning district as the number of facilities per square kilometre. In calculating this measure, all facilities within a one-block radius of the perimeter of a tract or district were included. This measure recognizes that facilities in close proximity to a tract or district may have as strong an impact as those facilities located within the defined boundaries. A limit of one block was selected because we have already demonstrated that within this distance negative attitudes toward facilities were most intense (see chapter 8). Because of the relatively large number of census tracts and planning

[5] A fuller account of the analysis undertaken in this section is reported in Hughes (1980).

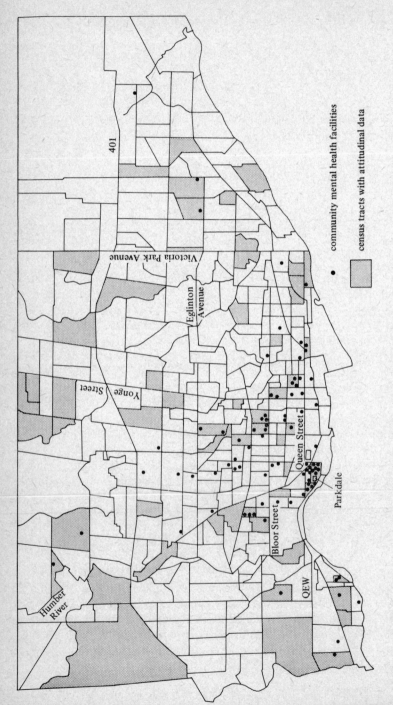

Figure 10.1. Distribution of community mental health facilities and census tracts. (Source: Hughes, 1980, page 33.)

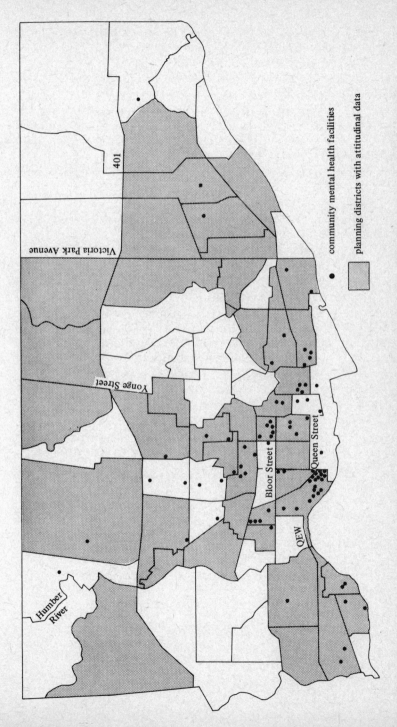

Figure 10.2. Distribution of community mental health facilities and planning districts. (Source: Hughes, 1980, page 34.)

districts with no facilities, the facility concentration values were grouped
into four separate categories: zero, low, moderate, and high (table 10.6).
The lower concentration values for planning districts reflects their larger
area. It is worthwhile noting that variations in facility type were ignored
in calculating the concentration index. It could be argued that differential
weightings should be assigned to different facility types based upon their
visibility and expected impact (compare chapters 2 and 8). This was not
attempted, however, because of the uncertainty involved in calculating a
weighting measure that would accurately represent the impacts of the
differing facility types. Furthermore, a weighting factor was not considered
crucial in the Toronto context because the majority of facilities within the
city are residential and small-scale.

The socioeconomic variables were assembled from readily available data
in the 1976 Census of Canada and the Metropolitan Toronto Board Land-
Use Directory. Variables were selected to represent the major social and
physical characteristics which previous studies have shown to be significant
in determining community response to mental health facilities (see section
10.2). These variables are: socioeconomic status, community stability,
density, land use, demographic structure, and community homogeneity
(table 10.7).

The relationship between facility concentration and neighbourhood
characteristics was examined by use of an analysis of variance for the
three levels of geographic scale: census tract, planning districts with
survey data, planning districts without survey data (that is, only socioenvironmental data). Seven variables are consistently related to facility
concentration for all levels of analysis (table 10.7): population density,
percentage of single individuals over fifteen years of age, percentage of
single-person households, percentage of detached buildings, percentage of

Table 10.6. Definition of facility concentration categories.

Geographic unit	Concentration category	Number of facilities	Concentration values
Census tracts	zero	30	0·00
	low	11	0·01–1·49
	moderate	8	1·50–5·99
	high	8	6·00–21·00
Planning districts (attitudinal/socio- environmental data)	zero	13	0·00
	low	13	0·01–0·49
	moderate	10	0·50–1·99
	high	6	2·00–6·00
Planning districts (socioenvironmental data only)	zero	36	0·00
	low	18	0·01–0·49
	moderate	12	0·50–1·99
	high	9	2·00–6·00

children under six years of age, percentage commercial land use, and ethnic diversity. The density variables are the only measures of facility concentration significant at all three levels of analysis. Demographic structure and community homogeneity are the only other dimensions which demonstrate relatively consistent relationships with facility concentration at all geographic scales. Family status and stage in the life cycle are significantly related to facility concentration, and detailed analysis confirms that areas of zero and low facility concentration tend to have greater numbers of children and fewer single people. In addition, greater ethnic diversity is found in areas of moderate and high facility concentration (Hughes, 1980, chapter 5). The relative inconsistency in the other socioeconomic categories is probably related to the variation in geographic scale of analysis.

A stepwise discriminant analysis was undertaken to determine the appropriate function to predict facility concentration. The results of the analysis of census tract data indicate that five socioeconomic variables made significant contributions to the discriminant functions. These variables, in order of inclusion, are: population density, percentage male population, percentage commercial land use, ethnic diversity, and percentage of population with some university education (table 10.8). The discriminant coefficients show that the first function is defined by a combination of all five variables. The second function is defined by a combination of population density and percentage male population as one pole, and by a combination of commercial land use, ethnic diversity, and university education as the other.

According to this analysis, census tracts with high facility concentration are characterized by high population densities, high percentage male population, high percentage commercial land use, high ethnic diversity, and a high percentage of the population with some university education. The distinction appearing here is between congested, diverse areas (census tracts with high facility concentration) and uncrowded, homogenous areas (tracts with low facility concentration). The contribution of the variables to the second function allows a further distinction to be drawn between areas of moderate and high facility concentration. Moderately concentrated areas are census tracts with relatively high levels of ethnic diversity, commercial land use, and university educated individuals. Highly concentrated areas are tracts with high population densities and male population. The distinction suggested here is between inner-city neighbourhoods (high concentration) and surrounding, low-status residential areas (moderate concentration).

Two significant discriminant functions emerge from the analysis of planning districts (table 10.9). The first function most clearly differentiates the zero and low areas from the moderate and high concentration areas. Planning districts with high facility concentrations are characterized by high population densities, high unemployment rates, greater ethnic

Table 10.7. Analysis of variance of socioeconomic variables.

Variable category	Independent variables	Level of analysis[a]		
		census tract	planning district (with attitudinal data)	planning district
Socioeconomic	mean income	3·0951***	1·9880	5·2654**
	percentage population with less than grade 9 education	1·8603	2·7577	12·3358*
	percentage population with some university education	2·7864***	1·8413	3·4404***
	house value	0·7397	0·7116	2·6932
	cash rent	2·4414	2·6166	9·1571*
Community stability	percentage population living in detached dwellings	3·8107***	11·7209*	20·0820*
	percentage population who are owner-occupiers	2·4684	7·3547*	10·6714*
	percentage population unemployed	2·3505	18·1560*	11·0415*
	percentage migrant population	0·5710	2·9009***	3·4728***
Density	population density	8·7313*	22·1094*	17·1197*
	percentage single-person households	3·9969**	6·3039*	7·5512*
	persons per household	1·1946	1·8007	1·3649
Land use	percentage commercial	4·3681**	3·1249***	7·5206*
	percentage industrial	0·4590	2·0364	3·8430***
	percentage residential	0·3884	1·2527	1·5292
	percentage industrial	0·6997	3·6653***	7·6476
Demographic structure	percentage male population	4·2980**	1·4084	2·5956
	percentage population single and over 15 years of age	8·3080*	11·2253*	13·5804*

percentage population under 15 years of age	3·1587***	3·5821	2·0514
percentage population under 6 years of age	2·7076***	3·1034	2·8201***
percentage population 18–25 years of age	1·9075	7·3164*	10·4693*
percentage population over 65 years of age	1·0236	1·6928	1·0510
Community homogeneity: ethnic diversity	3·1461***	9·2501*	13·7636*
percentage English-speaking population	1·7169	4·4174**	12·6912*

[a] Entries are F-values.
* Significant at the 0·001 level; ** significant at the 0·01 level; *** significant at the 0·05 level.

diversity, and a low percentage of children under six years of age. Areas of low facility concentration have the opposite traits. The contribution of the variables to the second function discriminates between zero and low concentration areas. On this function, the former exhibit high migration rates, and the latter have greater numbers of single-person households and young children. This suggests that areas of zero concentration are newly developed communities populated by families with older children. In low concentration areas, the neighbourhoods are older with a greater variation in available housing types. These areas have a greater preponderance of new families with young children.

Finally, the expansion of the discriminant analysis to include all the planning districts in the entire Metropolitan Toronto area substantially increases the number of zero concentration (suburban) areas, and their impact upon the results is evident. Seven variables contribute to only one significant discriminant function (table 10.10), but only two variables—population density and ethnic diversity—were significant in previous analyses. Four of the five remaining variables are all indicative of characteristics strongly associated with suburban areas, that is, low industrial

Table 10.8. Socioenvironmental variables (census tract)—discriminant function statistics.

Standardized coefficients	Function 1	Function 2
Population density	−0·57	0·44
Percentage male population	−0·48	0·68
Percentage commercial land use	−0·41	−0·49
Ethnic diversity	−0·32	−0·45
Percentage population with some university education	−0·53	−0·51
Wilks lambda	0·37*	0·72***

* Significant at the 0·001 level; *** significant at the 0·05 level.

Table 10.9. Socioenvironmental variables (planning district)—discriminant function statistics.

Standardized coefficients	Function 1	Function 2
Population density	0·68	−0·90
Percentage single-person households	−0·07	1·76
Percentage unemployed	0·52	0·38
Percentage migrant population	0·09	−1·13
Percentage population under six years of age	−0·58	1·70
Ethnic diversity	0·45	0·80
Wilks lambda	0·09**	0·45**

** Significant at the 0·01 level.

land use, low percentage single individuals over fifteen years of age, low
percentage of adults with less than grade nine education, and high numbers
of children between eighteen and twenty-five years of age. Only mean
income (the weakest contributing variable) is inconsistent with this pattern.

Table 10.10. Socioenvironmental variables (all planning districts)—discriminant
function statistics.

Standardized coefficients	Function 1
Population density	−0·40
Percentage population single and over 15 years of age	−0·55
Mean income	−0·25
Percentage population with less than grade nine education	−0·47
Percentage population 18–25 years of age	0·45
Percentage industrial	−0·30
Ethnic diversity	−0·45
Wilks lambda	0·19*

* Significant at the 0·001 level.

10.3.2 Comparison with predicted distribution

Density and community homogeneity measures were identified to be the
most important factors related to facility concentration. Other important
variables were: percentage single individuals over fifteen years of age,
percentage male population, percentage of children under six years of age,
and percentage unemployed. The relationships of these variables to the
differing levels of facility concentration were consistent with a priori
expectations. The higher concentration groups were characterized by
higher population densities, greater ethnic diversity, higher proportions of
the population that are single or male, higher rates of unemployment, and
fewer young children. The distinctiveness of these groups relative to these
characteristics was more apparent at the planning district level. The zero
and low concentration areas had very similar socioeconomic characteristics.
These areas were seen to have lower population densities and greater ethnic
homogeneity.

An informal comparison of the profiles of neighbourhoods with existing
concentrations of Toronto facilities and the profiles of accepting and
rejecting neighbourhoods provokes some interesting speculation (tables
10.5 and 10.11). First, there is a degree of overlap between the social
and physical characteristics of those neighbourhoods which are potentially
accepting of facilities and those with *high to moderate concentrations* of
existing facilities; these are high density, mixed land-use areas with few
children. Similarly, potentially *rejecting* neighbourhoods are similar to

those with existing *low to zero concentrations*; they are stable, child-
oriented, residential areas. However, we cannot (at the moment)
accept the hypothesis that the existing pattern of high and low facility
concentrations in Toronto corresponds to the patterns of neighbourhood
acceptance and rejection. This is because (1) there is no complete historical
record of attempted sitings of mental health facilities in Toronto, (2) the
history of conflict over sitings has included rejecting behaviour in areas
with existing high to moderate facility concentrations, (3) a range of
intervening variables has not been taken into account in our analysis (see
earlier in this section), and (4) there are conceptual problems with the
measures of 'acceptance' we have adopted (they do not, for instance, take
account of 'nonrejecting' behaviour, nor the powerlessness of some
neighbourhoods to achieve successful exclusionary outcomes). For the
moment at least, these fascinating dimensions of our analysis must remain
at the level of speculation, and serve as a stimulus to further research.

Table 10.11. Profiles of neighbourhood characteristics of areas with differing
concentrations of mental health facilities.

Level of facility concentration			
high	moderate	low	zero
Few children[a]		many children[b]	many children[c]
Well-educated[a]	well-educated[a]	low education level[a]	low education[c]
Large male population[a]		small male population[a]	
Ethnic diversity[a]	ethnic diversity[a]	ethnic homogeneity[a]	
		few single-person households[b]	
			high migration[c]
High density[a]		low density[a]	
Commercial land use[a]	commercial land use[a]	low commercial land use[a]	low industrial land use[c]

[a] Characteristic derived from table 10.8.
[b] Characteristic derived from table 10.9.
[c] Characteristics derived from table 10.10.

Conclusions

Our concern in this book has been to understand community attitudes toward the mentally ill and mental health facilities. In particular, we have tried to explain the attitudinal and behavioural responses of local residents to neighbourhood-based mental health care, to determine the impact of mental health facilities upon host communities, and to develop profiles of accepting and rejecting neighbourhoods for planning purposes. This final chapter briefly summarizes the major tenor of our findings with respect to these three themes, and examines their implications for the planning of mental health care.

11.1 Summary of major findings
Mental health facilities are typically regarded as 'noxious' facilities. These are often needed in communities, but are often rejected by residents adjacent to potential sites. Whenever conflict has arisen over the siting of such controversial facilities, events tend to be dominated by two phenomena: first, the political process through which the locational decision is resolved; and, second, the attitudes and behaviours of the opposing community. In this study, we have approached these issues through the analysis of public facility location theory and the theory of attitudes and behaviour (chapter 2).

The background to our study is the community mental health care 'revolution'. Historical evidence shows that the mentally ill have always been isolated and excluded from mainstream society, despite constant change in the philosophies of care (chapter 3). The current move away from asylum-based institutional care has created a new 'asylum without walls' in many inner-city neighbourhoods. A fundamental point of departure in our inquiry has been that such neighbourhoods are typically unprepared for the influx of ex-psychiatric patients, who may find themselves in, but not part of, a community.

We believe, with many others, that the successful resocialization of the mentally ill depends upon their acceptance by residents of the 'host' community. There has been a significant improvement in public awareness of mental illness since the Second World War. Our review (chapter 4) also suggests a fair degree of community tolerance of the mentally ill, but that this tolerance is fragile. In any specific setting, it can be fractured by the interplay of such factors as patient characteristics and behaviour, aspects of the treatment setting, and the personal characteristics of the nonuser. We tried to develop a model which would take account of these complex interactions (section 2.3). Neighbourhood acceptance or rejection was viewed as the outcome of an extended sequence of events. First in this sequence is a set of three 'external' factors determining community predispositions toward mental health care: characteristics of the facility and its user, the personality and status of the observer, and the social and physical characteristics of the host neighbourhood. These factors come together to determine a set of beliefs about the mentally ill, the facility in question, and the neighbourhood. Such beliefs are translated into attitudes and behavioural intentions which ultimately lead to action which is the basis of facility acceptance or rejection.

To test this model of community response, a survey of 1090 Toronto households was undertaken (chapter 5). Initially, two important sets of scales were developed. The first characterized community beliefs about mental illness along four dimensions: authoritarianism, emphasizing the need for coercive handling of the mentally ill; social restrictiveness, supportive of isolating the mentally ill from the rest of society; benevolence, a sympathetic view of the need to care for society's disabled; and a community mental health ideology, which summarized a procommunity, anti-institutional bias toward mental health care (section 6.1). The second set of scales were developed to represent respondents' beliefs about the suitability of their neighbourhood as a facility location. Six dimensions of neighbourhoods were addressed: activity, design, safety, predictability, integration, and evaluation (section 6.2).

Our test of the community response model (chapter 7) supported its general logic. Study data confirmed the relationship between external variables and beliefs, between beliefs and attitudes, and between attitudes and behavioural intentions. The final link in the model, between actual behaviour and intentions, remained untested because of low response rates in that part of the survey. Of the three sets of external variables—facility, neighbourhood, and personal characteristics—the group of personal factors was the most important predictor of beliefs about mental illness. Especially important were three demographic variables (age, sex, and number of children), two socioeconomic factors (education and tenure), and two belief measures (church attendance and familiarity with mental illness). Beliefs about mental illness were more important than facility or neighbour-hood characteristics in determining community attitudes toward the mental health facility. This seems to confirm the view that attitudes toward community-based mental health care are primarily a response to facility users. Finally, we found that those respondents rating facilities as undesirable are more likely to engage in opposition, and that the degree of commitment is directly related to the strength of the negative attitude. Thus, the link between attitudes and behavioural intentions was substantiated.

Next, we wanted to establish the exact sources of community opposition to mental health facilities. What, precisely, were residents objecting about? and, how limited was the geographical extent of these impacts and the opposition they generated? (chapter 8). It is somewhat surprising that only one-quarter of our respondents anticipated a negative impact following the opening of a facility. Those who were aware of a facility tended to be more tolerant in evaluating impact. Residents' fears are most commonly focussed on users' behaviour, property value decline, and increased traffic volumes. Negative attitudes are strongest within one block of a facility, but beyond six blocks the impact of a facility appears to be effectively neutralized. Attitudes are also affected by the type of facility in question, especially whether it is residential or nonresidential in operation. One of our most significant discoveries in this part of the work was that actual behavioural adjustments in response to a facility were very limited in scope and magnitude.

We thought it worthwhile to conduct an in-depth analysis of the most common complaint levelled against mental health facilities—the anticipated property value decline (chapter 9). In the five Toronto neighbourhoods we examined, there was no significant change in the volume of sales before, during or after a facility's opening. A small reduction in property values noted in some neighbourhoods could not be conclusively linked to the facility. Market movements seem to be due to such traditional factors as neighbourhood desirability and the characteristics of the housing unit being sold.

Finally, we attempted to develop profiles of accepting and rejecting neighbourhoods in order to facilitate planning for mental health facility locations (chapter 10). Accepting neighbourhoods are typically inner-city areas of relatively high population. Rejecting neighbourhoods tend to be stable, low-density residential areas with many young children.

11.2 Planning for community mental health facility location
It is difficult to distil the policy implications out of such a manifestly complex phenomenon as community attitudes toward mental health care. At the risk of oversimplifying, we conclude that the Toronto sample demonstrates a relatively high degree of tolerance toward the mentally ill. Opposition is apparently confined to a small (but potentially vocal) minority, who are concerned mainly about the behavioural characteristics of the facility users. Other concerns, however legitimately felt, tend to be ill-informed (for example, the expectation of increased traffic volumes). Extensive media coverage of the volume, extent, and successes of community opposition might distort the wider picture of community tolerance; it is certainly true that the widespread reports of opposition are almost never balanced by reports of successful facility openings.

This information is important in planning the future of community mental health. The movement out of the institution, and into local communities, is likely to continue unabated. This is not only the case for mental health care, but also for many other service-dependent populations including criminal offenders, the elderly, mentally retarded, and physically disabled. The following issues of policy and politics therefore have ramifications which transcend the limits of this book.

1. *There is a continuing need to improve public awareness and education regarding the mentally ill.* Such a campaign should capitalize upon the

apparently high degree of existing community tolerance. It should especially address the facts of mental illness and the purposes of deinstitutionalization. In any potential siting conflict, an awareness program should explain the exact nature of a facility and its users, clarifying the false expectations of many communities regarding the impact of a facility (for example, on property values). Two findings from our study suggest that an educational campaign will increase community acceptance of mental health facilities, namely the positive effect of familiarity with mental illness on attitudes toward the mentally ill and in turn the strong relationship between these attitudes and reaction to facilities. We recognize that the existing level of community tolerance comprises a large body of neutral opinion both toward facilities and toward potential users. An important aim of any educational program, therefore, is to translate this nonopposition into positive support which is required if community-based facilities are to achieve the resocialization objectives underlying community mental health care.

2. *The costs and benefits of a decentralized system of mental health care have to be assessed.* There are two parts to this problem: (a) continued efforts toward a geographically dispersed facility system can be justified on three grounds: to ensure access to care, to ease the burden of care throughout the community being served, and to provide a variety of choice in residential settings for former psychiatric patients. All three objectives would tend to 'undo' the ghetto and prevent the further saturation of residential neighbourhoods. (b) However, such a policy of decentralization needs to be balanced by a consideration of the positive benefits of the ghetto. This client viewpoint on posthospital life is something we have not addressed in this book. Many studies have suggested that the ghetto is, in fact, a highly supportive environment for the ex-patient. Before dismantling it, for whatever reasons, we need to be absolutely clear about how this would affect the coping capacities of the discharged patient.

Moreover, a vital issue in any decision or decentralization is the potential reaction to facilities in communities which at present have not had to accept them. The profiles of acceptance and rejection from our analysis indicate that the existing distribution of facilities probably corresponds quite closely with spatial variations in community tolerance across the urban area. Attempts to achieve a more equal distribution of facilities is likely, therefore, to create more opposition than has been experienced to date. The extent to which educational efforts can offset and overcome negative attitudes is uncertain, but has to be considered in evaluating the costs and benefits of dismantling the ghetto.

3. *It is important to recognize and to concede legitimate community fears about a potential facility.* If people are frightened about 'risky' (that is, potentially dangerous and unpredictable) people being introduced into their neighbourhoods, then efforts should be made to allay these fears.

Many more hospital patients are now being discharged, and the probability of an incident occurring necessarily increases. The onus in this situation is upon the professionals to develop a responsible aftercare and supervisory program for discharged patients. The likelihood of such a program increasing the host community's willingness to accept the location of a facility is supported by the study findings. A significant percentage of respondents qualified their opinion about a facility in their neighbourhood on the basis of the level and quality of patient supervision.

4. *The role of the architecture and design of mental health facilities in community acceptance needs to be assessed.* Our study suggests that the impact of the facility itself is of minor importance in shaping community attitudes. The strongest evidence of this is the low level of public awareness of existing facilities. We suggest that a major reason for the lack of awareness is the fact that many facilities are effectively invisible because they are housed within existing buildings, whether residential or institutional. There seems good reason to maintain this policy in the hope of minimizing neighbourhood disruption through facility introduction. However, other studies have indicated that minor design concessions can significantly influence the degree of community acceptance. Such concessions have included building a screening wall, enlarging internal lobbies, and ensuring structural renovation. These contradictory experiences warrant fuller attention, because community acceptance may be facilitated, and such architectural and design modifications seem a small price to pay to ensure care of our disabled.

References

Adorno T W, Frenkel-Brunswick E, Levinson D J, Sanford R N, 1950 *The Authoritarian Personality* (Harper and Row, New York)

Ajzen I, Fishbein M, 1980 *Understanding Attitudes and Predicting Social Behaviour* (Prentice-Hall, Englewood Cliffs, NJ)

Alexander C, 1964 *Notes on the Synthesis of Form* (Harvard University Press, Cambridge, MA)

Allderidge P, 1979 "Hospitals, madhouses and asylums: cycles in the care of the insane" *British Journal of Psychiatry* **134** 321-334

Armstrong B, 1976 "Preparing the community for the patient's return" *Hospital and Community Psychiatry* **27** 349-356

Austin M, Smith T, Wolpert J, 1970 "The implementation of controversial facility complex programs" *Geographical Analysis* **2** 315-329

Aviram U, Segal S, 1973 "Exclusion of the mentally ill" *Archives of General Psychiatry* **29** 126-131

Aviram U, Syme S L, Cohen J B, 1976 "The effect of policies and programs on reduction of mental hospitalization" *Social Science and Medicine* **10** 571-577

Bach L, 1980 "Locational models for systems of private and public facilities based on concepts of accessibility and access opportunity" *Environment and Planning A* **12** 301-320

Baker F, Schulberg H, 1967 "The development of a community mental health ideology scale" *Community Mental Health Journal* **3** 216-225

Bassuk E L, Gerson S, 1978 "Deinstitutionalization and mental health services" *Scientific American* **238**(2) 46-53

Beigel A, Levinson A I (Eds), 1972 *The Community Mental Health Center: Strategies and Programs* (Basic Books, New York)

Bigman D, ReVelle C, 1978 "The theory of welfare considerations in public facility location problems" *Geographical Analysis* **10** 229-240

Bigman D, ReVelle C, 1979 "An operational approach to welfare considerations in applied public facility location models" *Environment and Planning A* **11** 83-95

Blishen B R, McRoberts H A, 1976 "A socio-economic index for occupations in Canada" *Canadian Review of Sociology and Anthropology* **13** 71-79

Boeckh J, 1980 *Neighbourhood Effects of Community Mental Health Facilities* MA Thesis, Department of Geography, McMaster University, Hamilton, Ontario

Boeckh J L, Dear M, Taylor S M, 1980 "Property value effects of mental health facilities" *Canadian Geographer* **24**(3) 270-285

Bogardus E S, 1933 "A social distance scale" *Sociology and Social Research* **17** 265-271

Bord R, 1971 "Rejection of the mentally ill: continuities and further developments" *Social Problems* **18** 496-509

Breslow S, 1976 "The effect of siting group homes on the surrounding environments" unpublished paper, School of Architecture and Urban Planning, Princeton University, Princeton, NJ

Calvo A B, Marks D H, 1973 "Location of health care facilities: an analytical approach" *Socio-Economic Planning Sciences* **7** 407-422

Castells M, 1978 *City, Class and Power* (Macmillan, London)

Clare A, 1976 *Psychiatry in Dissent* (Tavistock Publications, London)

Clark A W, Binks N M, 1966 "Relation of age and education to attitudes toward mental illness" *Psychological Reports* **19** 649-650

Clark G, Dear M, 1978 "The state in capitalism and the capitalist state" discussion paper, Department of City and Regional Planning, Harvard University, Cambridge, MA; reprinted 1981 in *Urbanization and Urban Planning in Capitalist Society* Eds M Dear, A Scott (Methuen, London) pp 45-61

Cohen J, Struening E L, 1962 "Opinions about mental illness in the personnel of two large mental hospitals" *Journal of Abnormal and Social Psychology* **64** 349-360

Cohen J, Struening E L, 1963 "Opinions about mental illness: mental hospital occupational profiles and profile clusters" *Psychological Reports* **12** 111-145

Cohen J, Struening E L, 1964 "Opinions about mental illness: hospital social atmosphere profiles and their relevance to effectiveness" *Journal of Consulting Psychology* **28** 291-298

Cohen J, Struening E L, 1965 "Opinions about mental illness: hospital differences in attitude for eight occupational groups" *Psychological Reports* **17** 25-26

Community Mental Health Center Project, 1972 *Community Health Center Project* three volumes, Department of Health, Government of Canada, Ottawa (Queen's Printer, Ottawa)

Craik K, 1971 "The environmental adjective check list" Institute of Personality Assessment and Research, University of California, Berkeley, CA

Cumming E, Cumming J, 1957 *Closed Ranks: An Experiment in Mental Health* (Harvard University Press, Cambridge, MA)

D'Arcy C, 1976 "The manufacturing and obsolescence of madness" *Social Science and Medicine* **10** 5-13

Dear M, 1976 "Spatial externalities and locational conflict" *London Papers in Regional Science 7: Alternative Frameworks for Analysis* Eds D B Massey, P W J Batey (Pion, London) pp 152-167

Dear M, 1977 "Impact of mental health facilities on property values" *Community Mental Health Journal* **13** 150-157

Dear M, 1978 "Planning for mental health care: a reconsideration of public facility location theory" *International Regional Science Review* **3** 93-111

Dear M, 1981 "Social and spatial reproduction of the mentally ill" in *Urbanization and Urban Planning in Capitalist Society* Eds M Dear, A J Scott (Methuen, London) pp 481-500

Dear M, Fincher R, Currie L, 1977 "Measuring the external effects of public programs" *Environment and Planning A* **9** 137-147

Dear M, Taylor S M, Hall G B, 1980 "External effects of mental health facilities" *Annals, Association of American Geographers* **70**(3) 342-352

Dear M, Wolch J, 1980 "The optimal assignment of human service clients to treatment settings" in *Locational and Environmental Context of Elderly Population* Ed. S M Golant (V H Winston, New York)

Delottinville C B, 1976 "The asylum for the insane: a study of the history of institutional care and treatment of the mentally ill in Ontario 1820-1900" research report, School of Social Work, McGill University, Montreal

Deutsch A, 1949 *The Mentally Ill in America* (Columbia University Press, New York)

Dohrenwend D P, Chin-Shong E, 1967 "Social status and attitudes toward psychological disorder: the problem of tolerance and deviance" *American Sociological Review* **32** 417-433

Dökmeci V F, 1979 "A multiobjective model for regional planning of health facilities" *Environment and Planning A* **11** 517-525

Donzelot J, 1979 *The Policing of Families* (Pantheon Books, New York)

Ellsworth R B, 1965 "A behavioural study of staff attitudes toward mental illness" *Journal of Abnormal Psychology* **70** 194-200

Farina A, Felnen R, Bourdreau L, 1973 "Relation of workers to male and female mental patient job applicants" *Journal of Consulting and Clinical Psychology* **41** 363-372

Fischer E, 1971 "Who volunteers for companionship with mental patients? A study of attitude-belief-intention relationships" *Journal of Personality* **39** 552-563

Fishbein M, Ajzen I, 1972 "Attitudes and opinions" *Annual Review of Psychology* **23** 487-544

Fishbein M, Ajzen I, 1975 *Belief, Attitude, Intention and Behaviour: An Introduction to Theory and Research* (Addison Wesley, Reading, MA)

Foucault M, 1973 *Madness and Civilization: A History of Madness in the Age of Reason* (Vintage Books, New York)

Fournet G, 1967 "Cultural correlates with attitudes, perception, knowledge and reported incidence of mental disorders" *Dissertation Abstracts* **28**(1B) 339

Fracchia J, Canale D, Cambria E, Fuest E, Sheppard C, 1976 "Public views of ex-mental patients: a note on perceived dangerousness and unpredictability" *Psychological Reports* **38** 495-498

Fracchia J, Pintry J, Cravello J, Sheppard C, Merlin S, 1972 "Comparison of inter-correlations of scale scores from the opinions about mental illness scale" *Psychological Reports* **30** 149-150

Freedman A M, 1967 "Historical and political roots of the community mental health centers act" *American Journal of Orthopsychiatry* **37** 487-494

Freeman H E, 1961 "Attitudes toward mental illness among relatives of former patients" *American Sociological Review* **26** 59-66

Freestone R, 1977 *Public Facility Location* Exchange Bibliography 1211, Council of Planning Librarians, Monticello, IL

Gilbert D C, Levinson D J, 1956 "Ideology, personality and institutional policy in the mental hospital" *Journal of Abnormal and Social Psychology* **53** 263-271

Gingell T, Papp J, Szuch L, Whyte A, 1975 "Attitudes and intensity of reactions toward the location of urban public facilities" unpublished paper, Department of Geography, McMaster University, Hamilton, Ontario

Goffman E, 1961 *Asylums* (Doubleday Anchor, New York)

Gonen A, 1977 "Community support system for mentally handicapped adults: an alternative to spatially distributed human service facilities" discussion paper 96, Regional Science Research Institute, University of Pennsylvania, Philadelphia, PA

Goodale T, Wickware J, 1979 "Group homes and property values in residential areas" *Plan Canada* **19** 154-163

Gough H G, Heilbrun A B, 1965 *The Adjective Check List Manual* Consulting Psychologists Press, Palo Alto, CA

Greenblat M, 1978 *Psychopolitics* (Grune and Stratton, New York)

Greer-Wootten B, Patel B, 1976 "A social class stratification of Toronto CMA 1971" research report, Survey Research Centre, York University, Downsview, Ontario

Grob G N, 1973 *Mental Institutions in America: Social Policy to 1875* (Free Press, New York)

Hall G B, 1980 *Individual Responses to Community Mental Health Care* doctoral dissertation, Department of Geography, McMaster University, Hamilton, Ontario

Halpert H P, 1969 "Public acceptance of the mentally ill" *Public Health Reports* **84** 59-64

Hammer T, Horn E, Coughlin R, 1971 "The effect of a large urban park on real estate value" discussion paper 51, University of Pennsylvania, Regional Science Research Institute, Philadelphia, PA

Hanly J, 1970 *Health Services in Ontario* (Queen's Printer, Ottawa)

Harvey D W, 1973 *Social Justice and the City* (Edward Arnold, London)

Hillsman E L, Rushton S, 1976 "Solutions for multi-attribute location problems" unpublished paper, Department of Geography, University of Iowa, Iowa City, Iowa 52242

Hirsch J, Borowitz G, 1973 "The tyranny of treatment" paper read at the American Psychiatric Convention, Hawaii

Hodgart R L, 1978 "Optimizing access to public services: a review of problems, models and methods of locating central facilities" *Progress in Human Geography* **2** 17-48

Hodge D, Gatrell A, 1976 "Spatial constraint and the location of urban public facilities" *Environment and Planning A* **8** 215-230

Hodgson M J, 1978 "Toward a more realistic allocation in location-allocation: an interaction approach" *Environment and Planning A* **10** 1273-1285

Hollingshead A B, Redlich F C, 1958 *Social Class and Mental Illness* (John Wiley, New York)

Hughes R, 1980 *Spatial Concentration of Community Mental Health Facilities* MA thesis, Department of Geography, McMaster University, Hamilton, Ontario

Hurd H M (Ed.), 1973 *The Institutional Case of the Insane in the United States and Canada* four volumes (Arno Press, NY)

Isaak S, Taylor S M, Dear M, 1980 "Community mental health facilities in residential neighbourhoods" in *York University Geographical Monographs 8: Canadian Studies in Medical Geography* Ed. F E Barrett, Department of Geography, Downsview, Ontario, pp 231-256

Jessop R, 1977 "Recent theories of the capitalist state" *Cambridge Journal of Economics* **1** 353-374

Johnston R J, 1980 "Political geography without politics" *Progress in Human Geography* **4** 439-446

Jones K, 1972 *A History of the Mental Health Services* (Routledge and Kegan Paul, Henley-on-Thames, Oxon)

Joseph A, 1979 "The referral system as a modifier of distance decay effects in the utilization of mental health care services" *The Canadian Geographer* **23** 159-169

Klee G, Spiro E, Bahn A, Gorwitz K, 1967 "An ecological analysis of diagnosed mental illness in Baltimore" in *Psychiatric Epidemiology and Mental Health Planning* Eds R Monroe, C Klee, E Brody, psychiatric research report 22, American Psychiatric Association, Washington, DC

Klerman G L, 1977 "Better but not well: social and ethical issues in the deinstitutionization of the mentally ill" *Schizophrenia Bulletin* **3** 617-631

Knox P L, 1978 "The intraurban ecology of primary medical care: patterns of accessibility and their policy implications" *Environment and Planning A* **10** 415-435

LaFave H, Rootman I, Sydiaha D, Duckworth R, 1967 "The ethnic community and the definition of mental illness" *Psychiatric Quarterly* **41** 211-227

LaPiere R T, 1934 "Attitudes vs actions" *Social Forces* **13** 230-237

Lea A C, 1973 "Location-allocation systems: an annotated bibliography" discussion paper 13, Department of Geography, University of Toronto, Toronto, Ontario

Lemieux M, 1977 "One hundred years of mental health law in Ontario" unpublished paper, Hamilton Psychiatric Hospital, Hamilton, Ontario

Lemkau P, Crocetti S, 1962 "An urban population's opinion and knowledge about mental illness" *American Journal of Psychiatry* **118** 692-700

Lichfield N, 1970 "Evaluation methodology of regional plans" *Regional Studies* **4** 151-165

Linsky A, 1970 "Who shall be excluded: the influence of personal attributes to the mentally ill" *Social Psychiatry* **5** 166-171

Longwoods Research Group, 1980 *Development and Pretesting of a Public Education Programme on Group Homes* report to government of Ontario Department of Community and Social Services, Toronto, Ontario

McAllister D M, 1976 "Efficiency and equity in public facility location" *Geographical Analysis* **8** 47-63

McAllister D M, 1980 *Evaluation in Environmental Planning* (MIT Press, Cambridge, MA)

McGrew J C, Monroe C B, 1975 "Efficiency, equity and multiple facility location" *Proceedings, Association of American Geographers* **7** 142-146

MacLean U, 1969 "Community attitudes to mental illness in Edinburgh" *British Journal of Preventative and Social Medicine* **23** 45-52

Magaro P A, Gripp R, McDowell D J, 1978 *The Mental Health Industry: A Cultural Phenomenon* (Wiley Interscience, New York)

Massey D S, 1980 "Residential segregation and spatial distribution of a nonlabour force population: the needy, elderly and disabled" *Economic Geography* **56** 190–200

Mechanic D, 1969 *Mental Health and Social Policy* (Prentice-Hall, Englewood Cliffs, NJ)

Metropolitan Toronto Association for the Mentally Retarded, 1979 personal communication of unpublished data

Michelson W, 1970 *Man and His Urban Environment* (Addison-Wesley, Reading, MA)

Morrill R, 1974 "Efficiency and equity of optimum location models" *Antipode* **6** 179–190

Mumphrey A, Wolpert J, 1973 "Equity considerations and concessions in the siting of public facilities" *Economic Geography* **94** 109–121

National Institute of Mental Health, 1976 *Deinstitutionalization: A Sociological Perspective* National Institute of Mental Health, Washington, DC

Nunnally J, 1957 "The communication of mental health information: a comparison of experts and the public with news media presentations" *Behavioural Scientist* **2** 222

Nunnally J, 1961 *Popular Conceptions of Mental Health: Their Development and Change* (Holt, Rinehart and Winston, New York)

Nunnally J, 1967 *Psychometric Theory* (McGraw-Hill, New York)

Olives J, 1976 "The struggle against urban renewal in the Cité D'Aliarte" in *Urban Sociology: Critical Essays* Ed. C A Pickvance (Tavistock Publications, London) pp 174–197

Olmstead P, Durham K, 1976 "Stability of mental health attitudes: a semantic differential study" *Journal of Health and Social Behaviour* **17** 35–44

Olson M, 1965 *The Logic of Collective Action: Public Goods and the Theory of Groups* (Harvard University Press, Cambridge, MA)

Ontario Health Planning Task Force, 1974 *Report of the Health Planning Task Force* Ontario Government Publications, Toronto, Ontario

Ontario Ministry of Health, 1974 *Hospital Statistics* Ontario Government Publications, Toronto, Ontario

Osgood C E, Suci G J, Tannenbaum P H, 1957 *The Measurement of Meaning* (University of Illinois Press, Urbana, IL)

Page S, 1977 "The effects of mental illness label in attempts to obtain accommodation" *Canadian Journal of Behaviour Science* **9** 85–90

Papageorgiou G J, 1978 "Spatial externalities: Parts I and II" *Annals, Association of American Geographers* **68** 465–492

Peet R, 1975 "Inequality and poverty: a Marxist geographic approach" *Annals, Association of American Geographers* **65** 564–571

Phillips D C, 1963 "Rejection: a possible consequence of seeking help for mental disorders" *American Sociological Review* **28** 963–972

Phillips D L, 1964 "Rejection of the mentally ill: the influence of behaviour and sex" *American Sociological Review* **29** 679–687

Phillips D R, 1979 "Public attitudes to general practitioner services: a reflection of an inverse care law in intraurban primary medical care?" *Environment and Planning A* **11** 815–824

President's Commission on Mental Health, 1978 four volumes (US Government Printing Office, Washington, DC)

Rabkin J G, 1972 "Opinions about mental illness: a review of the literature" *Psychological Bulletin* **77** 153–171

Rabkin J G, 1974 "Public attitudes toward mental illness: a review of the literature" *Schizophrenia Bulletin* **1** 9-33

Rabkin J G, 1975 "The role of attitudes toward mental illness in evaluation of mental health programs" in *Handbook of Evaluation Research, Volume 2* Eds M Guttentag, E L Struening (Sage Publications, Beverley Hills, CA) pp 431-482

Rabkin J G, 1977 "Public attitudes about mental illness: literature review and recommendations" paper prepared for Task Panel on Public Attitudes and use of Media for Promotion of Mental Health, President's Commission on Mental Health, Washington, DC

Ramsey G V, Seipp M, 1948a "Attitudes and opinions concerning mental illness" *Psychiatric Quarterly* **22** 428-444

Ramsey G V, Seipp M, 1948b "Public opinions and information concerning mental health" *Journal of Clinical Psychology* **4** 397-406

Reiner T A, Wolpert J, 1981 "The non-profit sector in the metropolitan community" *Economic Geography* **57** 23-33

ReVelle C S, Marks D, Liebman J, 1970 "An analysis of private and public sector location models" *Management Science* **16** 692-708

ReVelle C S, Swain R W, 1970 "Central facilities location" *Geographical Analysis* **2** 30-42

Richman A, 1964 *Psychiatric Care in Canada: Extent and Results* (Queen's Printer, Ottawa)

Ring S, Chein L, 1970 "Attitudes toward mental illness and the use of caretakers in a black community" *American Journal of Orthopsychiatry* **40** 710-716

Rojeski P, ReVelle C S, 1970 "Central facilities location under an investment constraint" *Geographical Analysis* **2** 343-360

Rosen G, 1968 *Madness in Society* (Harper and Row, New York)

Rosenzweig N, 1975 *Community Mental Health Programs in England: An American View* (Wayne State University Press, Detroit, MI)

Rothenburg J, 1967 *Economic Evaluation of Urban Renewal* The Brookings Institute, Washington, DC

Rothman D J, 1971 *The Discovery of the Asylum: Social Order and Disorder in the New Republic* (Little, Brown, Boston, MA)

Rothman D J, 1980 *Conscience and Convenience: The Asylum and Its Alternatives in Progressive America* (Little, Brown, Boston, MA)

Rutman I, Piasecki J, Baron R, 1980, personal communication

Sarbin T R, Mancuso J C, 1972 "Paradigms and moral judgements: improper conduct is not a disease" *Journal of Consulting and Clinical Psychology* **39** 6-8

Schall L D, 1971 "A note on externalities and property valuation" *Journal of Regional Science* **11** 101-105

Scheff T, 1966 *Being Mentally Ill* (Aldine, Chicago, IL)

Scheff T, 1967 *Mental Illness and Social Progress* (Harper and Row, New York)

Schmedemann D A, 1979 "Zoning for the mentally ill: a legislative mandate" *Harvard Journal of Legislation* **16** 853-899

Schneider J B, Symons J C, 1971 "Regional health facility systems planning: an access-opportunity approach" discussion paper 68, Regional Science Research Institute, University of Pennsylvania, Philadelphia, PA

Schuler R E, Holahan W L, 1977 "Optimal size and spacing of public facilities in metropolitan areas" *Papers, Regional Science Association* **39** 137-156

Scott A J, 1980 *The Urban Land Nexus and the State* (Pion, London)

Scull A T, 1978 *Decarceration: Community Treatment of the Deviant—A Radical View* (Prentice-Hall, Englewood Cliffs, NJ)

See P, 1968 "The labelling and allocation of deviance in a southern state: a socio-logical theory" *Dissertation Abstracts* **29**(2A) 687-688

Segal S, Aviram U, 1978 *The Mentally Ill in Community-based Sheltered Care* (John Wiley, New York)

Segal S, 1978 "Attitudes toward the mentally ill: a review" *Social Work* **23** 211-217

Seley J E, 1981a "Introduction: new directions in public services" *Economic Geography* **57** 1-9

Seley J E (Ed.), 1981b "New directions in public services" *Economic Geography* **57**(1) special issue

Seley J E, 1981c "Targeting economic development: an examination of the needs of small businesses" *Economic Geography* **57** 34-51

Simon B, 1978 *Mind and Madness in Ancient Greece: The Classical Roots of Modern Psychiatry* (Cornell University Press, Ithaca, New York)

Smith C A, Smith C J, 1978 "Learned helplessness and preparedness in discharged mental patients" *Social Work Research and Abstracts* **14** 21-27

Smith C J, 1976a "Distance and the location of community mental health facilities: a divergent viewpoint" *Economic Geography* **52** 181-191

Smith C J, 1976b "Residential neighbourhoods as humane environments" *Environment and Planning A* **9** 585-597

Smith C J, Hanham R Q, 1981 "Proximity and the formation of public attitudes towards mental illness" *Environment and Planning A* **13** 147-165

Star S, 1955 *The Public's Ideas About Mental Illness* report, National Opinion Research Center, University of Chicago, Chicago, IL

Steiner P O, 1970 "The public sector and the public interest" in *Public Expenditures and Policy Analysis* Eds R H Haveman, J Margolis (Markham, Chicago, IL) pp 21-58

Stimson R J, 1980 "Spatial aspects of epidemiological phenomena and of the provision and utilization of health care services in Australia: a review of methodological problems and empirical analyses" *Environment and Planning A* **12** 881-907

Taylor S M, Breston B E, Hall F L, 1982 "The effect of road traffic noise on house prices" *Journal of Sound and Vibration* **80**(4) 523-541

Taylor S M, Dear M, 1981 "Scaling community attitudes toward the mentally ill" *Schizophrenia Bulletin* **7**(2) 225-240

Taylor S M, Dear M, Hall G B, 1979 "Attitudes toward the mentally ill and reactions to mental health facilities" *Social Science and Medicine* **13D** 281-290

Taylor S M, Hall F, 1977 "Factors affecting response to road noise" *Environment and Planning A* **9** 585-597

Teitz M, 1968 "Toward a theory of urban public facility location" *Papers, Regional Science Association* **21** 35-52

Thouez J P, 1975 "Idéntité, structure, signification des edifices de service public et compartements de migrants" bulletin de recherche 19, Départment de Géographie, Université de Sherbrooke, Québec

Toronto Real Estate Board, 1978 *House Price Trends: 1978 Edition* Toronto Real Estate Board, Toronto, Ontario

Tringo J L, 1970 "The hierarchy of preference toward disability groups" *The Journal of Special Education* **4** 295-306

Trute B, Segal S, 1976 "Census tract predictors and the social integration of sheltered care residents" *Social Psychiatry* **11** 153-161

Wagner J L, Falkson L M, 1975 "The optimal modal location of public facilities with price-sensitive demand" *Geographical Analysis* **7** 69-83

Webb E J, Campbell D T, Schwartz R D, Sechrest L, 1966 *Unobtrusive Measures: Nonreactive Research in the Social Sciences* (Rand McNally, Chicago, IL)

Weiss P, Macaulay J, Pincus A, 1966 "Geographic factors and the release of patients from state mental hospitals" *American Journal of Psychiatry* **123** 408-412

Western Institute for Research in Mental Health, 1967 *Planning, Programming and Design for the Community Mental Health Center* Mental Health Materials Center, NY

Whatley C, 1959 "Social attitudes toward discharged mental patients" *Social Problems* **6** 313-320

White A, 1979 "Accessibility and public facility location" *Economic Geography* **55** 18-35

Wicker A, 1969 "Attitudes versus actions: the relationship of verbal and overt behavioural responses to attitude objects" *Journal of Social Issues* **25** 41-78

Williams J I, Luterbach E J, 1976 "The changing boundaries of psychiatry in Canada" *Social Science and Medicine* **10** 15-22

Wolch J R, 1979 "Residential locations and the provision of human services" *Professional Geographer* **31** 271-276

Wolch J R, 1980 "Residential location of the service dependent poor" *Annals, Association of American Geographers* **70** 330-341

Wolch J R, 1981 "The location of service-dependent households in urban areas" *Economic Geography* **57** 52-67

Wolpert J, 1977 "Social income and the voluntary sector" *Papers, Regional Science Association* **39** 137-156

Wolpert J, 1978 *Group Homes for the Mentally Retarded and Investigation of Neighbouring Property Impacts* Woodrow Wilson School of Public and International Affairs, Princeton University, Princeton, NJ

Wolpert J, 1980 "The dignity of risk" *Transactions, Institute of British Geographers* new series **5** 391-401

Wolpert J, Dear M, Crawford R, 1975 "Satellite mental health facilities" *Annals, Association of American Geographers* **65** 24-35

Wolpert J, Wolpert E, 1976 "The relocation of released mental hospital patients into residential communities" *Policy Sciences* **7** 31-51

Wood P A, 1977 "Location theory and spatial analysis" *Progress in Human Geography* **1** 487-491

Wood P A, 1978 "Location theory and spatial analysis" *Progress in Human Geography* **2** 518-525

Wood P A, 1979 "Location theory and spatial analysis" *Progress in Human Geography* **3** 583-589

Woodward J, 1951 "Changing ideas on mental illness and its treatment" *Sociological Review* **16** 443-454

Woogh C M, Meier H M R, Eastwood M R, 1977 "Psychiatric hospitalization in Ontario: revolving door in perspective" *Canadian Medical Association Journal* **116** 876

Subject index

Asylum, history of 40–52
Attitudes
  and behaviour 24–25, 30, 63–65, 67
  community 18–25, 30–31
  formation 19–24, 30–31, 35, 65–66
  role 18–21
  theory 18, 21, 23, 25, 30, 35–36
  toward facilities 18–26, 79–80,
    107–115

Behaviour 19–21, 23–25, 31–32,
  115–117
  and attitudes 24–25, 30, 63–65, 67
  of community groups 33–35
  of the mentally ill 27, 54–56
  outcomes 18–21, 25, 32–35,
    115–117
Behavioural intentions 19–21, 23, 25,
  31–32, 35, 113–115, 123–124,
  127–132
Beliefs
  behavioural 20–22, 30
  measurement 22, 28–30, 60–63,
    66–67, 85–97
  neighbourhood 23, 27, 29–30, 92–97
  normative 20–22, 30–35
  role 19–21, 23–25, 27–31, 35
  scales
    authoritarianism 22, 28, 77–78,
      86–91, 102–111
    benevolence 22, 77–78, 86–91,
      102–111
    CMHI 62–63, 85–86, 97
    CMI 62, 86
    community mental health ideology
      23, 77–78, 86–91, 102–111
    OMI 62–63, 66, 85–86, 97
    social restrictiveness 22, 77–78,
      86–91, 102–111

Community 15–16, 51–52, 146
  acceptance and rejection 140–154
  mental health care 17, 46–52
  mental health centers (US) 47–50
  profiles of accepting and rejecting
    153–154, 163–164

Deinstitutionalization 46–52, 59

External effects 10–13, 15–16
  behavioural response 120–132
  neighbourhood-associated 15

External effects (continued)
  spatial externality field 121–122,
    124–132
  user-associated 15, 121–122
  see also mental health facilities
External variables 20–21, 23–29, 35,
  56–69, 98–107
  demographic characteristics 20, 23, 27,
    56–58, 101–107
  neighbourhood characteristics 25, 28,
    34–35
  personality traits 20, 23, 28, 102
  religion 102, 104–107
  situational factors 20–21, 58–59
  socioeconomic status 20, 27, 57–58,
    101–107

Ghettoization 13, 16, 168
Group homes 18–19, 20, 27

Land use 21, 23, 28, 129–132
Location 13–17
  as access 13–14, 16
  as externality 13, 15–16
  social context of 13, 16–17
Locational conflict 10, 15–16, 34, 51–52

Mental health facilities
  attitudes towards 18–25, 79–80,
    107–115, 121, 168–169
  awareness of 98–100, 123–126,
    131–132, 167–168
  beliefs about 22–23, 27, 30, 78–79,
    98–101, 107–108
  community response model 25–35,
    98–118
  congruence 23, 27, 30, 80, 111–113
  design 25, 27, 29
  external effects 18–19, 22, 27–29,
    35, 119–132
  impact of 122–124
  integration 28–29
  location 18–19, 29, 32, 34
  size 20–21, 25, 27, 29
  supervision 25, 27
  in Toronto 155–164
  type 25, 27, 126–127, 129–132
  users 13–17, 22–23, 25, 27, 121–124
Mental illness 27, 37–51
  explanations of 38–51
  labelling 54
  treatment 55–56